The
Enlightened
Diet

The Enlightened Diet

7 Weight-Loss Solutions *That* Nourish Body, Mind, *and* Soul

Deborah Kesten, MPH, and Larry Scherwitz, PhD

CELESTIAL ARTS
Berkeley | Toronto

Celestial Arts
an imprint of Ten Speed Press
PO Box 7123
Berkeley, California 94707
www.tenspeed.com

Distributed in Australia by Simon and Schuster Australia, in Canada by Ten Speed Press Canada, in New Zealand by Southern Publishers Group, in South Africa by Real Books, and in the United Kingdom and Europe by Publishers Group UK.

Book design by Chloe Rawlins

Library of Congress Cataloging-in-Publication Data
Kesten, Deborah, 1948–
  The enlightened diet : seven weight-loss solutions that nourish body, mind, and soul / Deborah Kesten and Larry Scherwitz.

     p. cm.

  Includes bibliographical references and index.

  Summary: "A guide to seven eating styles that put people at greater risk for overeating and weight gain, along with strategies for overcoming them and maintaining optimal weight"—Provided by publisher.

  ISBN-13: 978-1-58761-311-1
  ISBN-10: 1-58761-311-5

  1. Weight loss. 2. Reducing diets. 3. Nutrition. I. Scherwitz, Larry. II. Title.
  RM222.2.K48 2007
  613.2'5—dc22

                    2007023037

First printing, 2007
Printed in the United States of America

1 2 3 4 5 6 7 8 9 10 — 11 10 09 08 07

Contents

Acknowledgments

We are deeply grateful to friends and colleagues who have contributed to the rich repository of food and weight wisdom that forms *The Enlightened Diet*. Thank you all for sharing your reflections, knowledge, and insights:

To the team at *Explore: The Journal of Science and Healing*, an interdisciplinary journal that explores the healing arts, consciousness, spirituality, environmental issues, and basic science, as all these fields relate to health, for publishing our research on the seven eating styles and their link to overeating, overweight, and obesity.

To Larry Dossey, brilliant visionary, friend, colleague, and executive editor of *Explore*, for shining his intellectual and spiritual light on our work.

To David Riley, editor-in-chief of *Explore*, for his supportive editorial.

To Barbara Dossey, whose pioneering work in holistic health, and extensive and scholarly research in her exceptional book *Florence Nightingale: Mystic, Visionary, Healer*, has been an ongoing inspiration.

To Jo Ann Deck, publisher of Ten Speed Press, for her authentic love of literature and good books, and for her interest in, and understanding of, *The Enlightened Diet*; we are deeply grateful.

To Brie Mazurek, senior editor at Ten Speed Press: thank you for your insights; it's a pleasure to work with you.

To Brenda Knight, dear friend and award-winning author: heartfelt thanks for making all good things possible.

To Linda Roghaar, our literary agent: we're so glad you're a kindred spirit and book aficionado.

To friend and colleague Barbara Birsinger, for sharing her personal and professional knowledge about emotional eating.

To Keri Brenner, award-winning journalist and friend, for telling us about her experience with "sensory eating," and for her professional interest in our work as a path that leads to weight loss.

To Vinita Azarow, friend and "fellowette" food aficionado . . . aaahhhhh . . . your story about your after-school meals with Nonna, your Italian grandmother, warms the heart . . . always.

To Bruce Heller, dear friend and physician, who shares our interest in Integrative Medicine: we're so glad that you "grock" the concept of Enlightened Exercise and that you told us about your passion for, and personal experience with, movement and motion.

To Gerdi Weider, a brilliant and exceptional research scientist and friend, who told us about her reversing-heart-disease lifestyle research at the Preventive Medicine Research Institute in Sausalito, California, and lifestyle's link to weight.

To Bruce Milliman, friend and naturopathic physician: we appreciate your contribution about naturopathy's perspective on exercise.

To Sheila Quinn, friend and fresh food maker, for sharing her delicious recipes.

To Cassandra Vieten, brilliant psychologist, researcher, and writer: thank you for giving us insights into "negative affect."

To Meg Jordan, a like-minded medical anthropologist and health journalist, for her unique and personalized approach to movement, motion, and exercise.

To research scientist, naturopath, and friend Leanna Standish: thank you for your helpful suggestions about "molecules of emotion" and "healing environments."

To all those we have mentioned, please know that we are honored to have had the opportunity to talk with you and to learn from you. You so eloquently shared your wisdom, insights, and expertise about the multidimensional ways in which food heals. Because of you, we have learned much about the gift that is food. And because of you, the stream of nutritional and weight wisdom continues to flow.

And to all those who, by living the Enlightened Diet, bypass eating-by-number and instead contribute to the human longing to find meaning in meals.

When you look at nutrition from a purely scientific point of view, there is no place for consciousness. And yet, consciousness could be one of the crucial determinants of the metabolism of food itself.[1]

—Deepak Chopra, MD

Ancient Food Wisdom Meets Modern Nutritional Science

We are researchers who specialize in obesity, nutrition, lifestyle, and health. Throughout our careers, we have dedicated ourselves to discovering how lifestyle choices you make each day (such as diet, exercise, stress management, social support, etc.) can prevent, manage, or reverse chronic conditions ranging from overweight and obesity to heart disease and diabetes. Because being overweight or obese significantly increases your risk not only of developing a chronic condition but also of dying from it, we became deeply interested in creating an evidence-based, sustainable program to reduce the American girth. We were especially interested in this because, as we write, more than two-thirds of Americans are either overweight or obese, and for the first time in two centuries, the life expectancy of the younger generation is projected to be shorter than that of their parents because of the ever-growing number of overweight children and teens.

Because traditional dieting doesn't bring lasting weight loss for most people, we began our nutrition journey around the world by studying what *does* work—as a way of life and eating, not as a typical restrictive food regimen. We researched nutrition and food wisdom from Western nutritional science, as well as from cultures (such as the Mediterranean and French) that are naturally thinner and healthier. But we didn't stop there. We also investigated timeless food wisdom from Eastern healing systems, such as traditional Chinese medicine

(TCM), India's Ayurvedic principles, and Tibetan Medicine. Excited about our findings, we continued our exploration of ancient food wisdom and modern nutritional science by analyzing dietary guidelines from world religions and cultural traditions (such as the yoga diet and Native American food beliefs); they provided advice about optimal nutrition and eating centuries before science became the uncontested expert in the twentieth century. During our quest, to add even more substance and understanding to our odyssey, we spoke with, and interviewed, more than fifty scientists, religionists, and spiritual experts.[2]

Our inspiration for conducting such an extensive investigation about food, nutrition, and diet over the centuries was inspired by a comment our friend and colleague, Larry Dossey, MD, wrote in his book *Reinventing Medicine*: "In order to understand how healing happens, in the twenty-first century, we shall look not only at our atoms and molecules but at consciousness as well. In so doing, we shall reinvent medicine, adding ancient wisdom to modern science."[3] Surely, we thought, there is a lot to learn about time-tested food wisdom from our nutritional ancestors.

Our next step was to make sense of all we had discovered about how people and cultures worldwide have regarded, prepared, savored, and shared food for millennia as a vehicle for connecting to its deeper significance. A sampling: Judaism's dietary laws are designed to honor both animal- and plant-based food; Christians honor the Divine by connecting to Jesus Christ through the bread and wine of Holy Communion; yogis eat, in part, to enhance health and well-being through the life-giving qualities in food; Buddhists pursue enlightenment by bringing a meditative awareness to food; African Americans celebrate food, life, and friendship by "spicing" soul food with love and cooking from "feel"; Muslims honor food, family, and friendship as a gift from Allah; and the Japanese turn to tea to renew the spirit.

Sound Science, Weight Loss Success

When we stepped back to reflect on what each wisdom and cultural tradition had to tell us about optimal eating, we were excited to discern six perennial principles: fresh food, feelings, mindfulness, gratitude, love, and socializing. To make meaning of these themes, we turned them into guidelines, which to our amazement grew into a comprehensive program for biological, psychological, spiritual, and social nourishment—hence, our term "whole person nutrition."[4] Here are the guidelines:

1. Eat fresh whole foods in their natural state as often as possible.
2. Be aware of feelings before, during, and after eating.
3. Bring moment-to-moment nonjudgmental awareness to every aspect of the meal.
4. Appreciate food and its origins—from the heart.
5. Create union with the Divine by "flavoring" food with love.
6. Unite with others through food.

As researchers committed to sound science, we felt fervor about our discovery because these guidelines are consistent with what health professionals worldwide recommend, as do caring cooks and the millions of us who savor and enjoy good food. But would the guidelines weigh in with weight loss? Was there a link between them and optimal eating? Would *not* following the guidelines lead to overeating, and being overweight or obese?

To find out, we partnered with *Spirituality & Health* magazine. In its cover story on our integrative eating guidelines (we have since adopted the term "whole person nutrition" as more reflective of our program), readers were invited to take our e-course, called "the Enlightened Diet," on the *Spirituality & Health* website.[5] One caveat: to gain access to our interactive, six-week, eighteen-lesson e-course, participants would first have to complete our eighty-item whole person nutrition survey, as well as list their height and weight. All lessons were replete with information and coaching and opportunities to internalize and practice the whole person nutrition guidelines via workshop-like exercises, "nutritips," discussion groups, and a question-and-answer section.

Though not all of the 5,256 people who participated in our e-course filled out the questionnaire at the end of the intervention, we were still able to assess whether they made changes in whole person nutrition, their degree of change, and whether modifying what and how they ate was linked to weight loss. We were astounded and inspired by what we discovered next: seven eating styles emerged that were linked with overeating, overweight, and obesity. And then our findings got even more interesting: *those whose eating style score improved the most during the e-course, lost the most weight.* When we took a closer look, we realized that, together, the eating styles reveal a pattern. Like members of a family, each is independent, but they also work together as a team, with each one having the power to influence the others. Our core discovery, though, is simple and straightforward: the more people disregard the time-tested wisdom from world religions and cultural traditions, Eastern healing systems, and Western nutritional science, the more they are likely to overeat and be overweight and obese.

Because our research was both solid and groundbreaking, when it was published in the peer-reviewed medical journal *Explore: The Journal of Science and Healing,* the editor-in-chief, David Riley, MD, wrote in his editorial that "these results provide a fresh perspective on our epidemic of overeating, overweight, and obesity . . . that . . . could signal a paradigm shift in the field of nutrition."[6] And what is that shift? Our all-encompassing new view of nutrition not only gives us new insights into why we overeat, like a sweeping beam of light, but it also provides grounding and direction about what we can do to reduce our growing girth.

We are especially excited to share the seven eating styles with you because our research suggests that the problem is, in large part, due to a dynamic web of food-related choices, feelings, sensations, and social behaviors that *work together* to form a *syndrome* that leads to overeating, overweight, and obesity. As members of a family unit, all seven eating styles have a role to play. When practiced together, they hold the power to contribute to weight gain . . . if you don't know what to do about them. Throughout this book, we guide you through the antidotes to each eating style, so you can unlock the code to turning your biological, psychological, spiritual, or social nutrition trouble spots into weight loss success. Because the eating styles encompass whole person nutrition concepts, they reflect the original meaning of the word *diet* as a way of life. "When we are nourished this way," writes Riley, "we may not need to compensate with overeating and satiety."[7]

Haste Makes Waist

What do the seven eating styles mean to those of us who want to lose weight and keep it off? Our discovery of the seven eating styles, which forms the basis of the Enlightened Diet, reveals that previously unknown food and eating choices you make can put you at greater risk for overeating and ensuing overweight and obesity. When you identify your eating styles and realize how each contributes to your weight gain, you will be able to develop antidotes, thereby unlocking the code to taking control of your weight, and to staying slim for life.

There's a caveat, though: what *you* contribute to the Enlightened Diet is as important, if not more important, than the insights and information we provide. There are three requisites for you to be successful: (1) a firm commitment and decision to change your approach to food and eating; (2) a willingness to take the necessary time to make beneficial changes; and (3) a commitment to a heartfelt regard for food and all food-related activities.

We understand that, for many, finding and taking the time to make changes in your relationship to food and eating is a major challenge.

But the solution lies in the problem. In other words, it is a *perceived* lack of time, and living with a consciousness of time starvation, that is the root of our society's overeating and overweight epidemic; this is because lack of time results in turning to the time-saving shortcut of processed food and eating-on-the-run. But mechanization of food results in poorer nutrition, and it also disconnects us from the preparation that imbues food and eating with regard and meaning. In turn, when food is not fulfilling, we appreciate it less and often cope by eating more and more. In this way, the time we take with all activities related to food has a hidden and powerful benefit: it may actually help to modify some of the eating styles and some of their cousins, such as overwork, overscheduling, even a sense of spiritual starvation.

As you'll see, our research-based diet program gives you more than *what* to eat to lose weight and enhance your well-being; it also reveals science-based eating style secrets, specific guidelines, practical choices, recipes, and rituals, about *how* to eat to stay slim for life. With simple, but potent, step-by-step strategies, our comprehensive program gives you the foundation, solid structure, and tools to put the antidotes to the eating styles into action, so that you can attain and maintain optimal weight and well-being.

A Note to the Reader
Though we jointly collaborated in the research and development of this book, instances of the first person singular ("I") reflect Deborah's individual voice.

Chapter 1

Whole Person Nutrition

Research on optimal health suggests that we need a new . . .
kind of healthcare professional who can integrate the best of
alternative care with the best of conventional medicine, along
with psychological, social, and spiritual counseling skills.[1]

—Kenneth R. Pelletier, PhD, MD

The Enlightened Diet is unlike any other diet or weight loss program you have ever done. It is not a quick-fix diet as you know it. It is not about calorie counting, figuring fat, or watching your weight. It's not low-carb or high-protein, nor is it a restrictive regimen. We are not suggesting traditional, nonscientific approaches to eating and weight loss because, over the decades, we have learned that these approaches simply don't work. And the reason, we have discovered, is that they do not address the underlying reasons most of us overeat. In contrast, the Enlightened Diet is effective because it is the first comprehensive program that gives you a way of eating that addresses *all* of the biological, psychological, spiritual, and social reasons you overeat. In this way, the Enlightened Diet is actually an expression of the ancient, original meaning of *diet* in the best sense of the word: it's a way of life and eating that can lead you naturally to weight loss and wellness.

Why do we describe the Enlightened Diet as a way to live instead of as a restrictive, traditional diet? If your intention is to lose weight, and you stay with it, you'll accomplish this . . . but also much more: you'll reap the rewards of more balanced emotions, spiritual well-being, and social connection. We call these multidimensional ways in which the Enlightened Diet heals "whole person nutrition," because not only will you discover optimal eating strategies for weight loss, but we will also show you how to make the most of your meals so that "all of you" will be nourished each time you eat. In other words, as you become more and more successful on this program, the more you will feel fulfilled without overeating, while at the same time you will experience both weight loss and "wellness living." And there are other benefits. You can also expect to see a lessening of food- and diet-related symptoms linked to some chronic conditions such as heart disease, diabetes, and high blood pressure, as well as a reduction in stress, anxiety, and depression. At the same time, you will reap the rewards of connecting to the meaning in your meals, as well as to community, such as friends, family, and coworkers.

From Diet Despair to Enlightenment

"We have stopped our investigation of healing well short of its potential," writes Larry Dossey, MD, in *Reinventing Medicine.*[2] In the same way, we have traditionally limited much of our investigation about losing weight and keeping it off to a one-size-fits-all, overly simplified, calories in–calories out formula: to lose weight, conventional wisdom tells us, the calories you consume (energy in) must be fewer than the calories you expend (energy out); to maintain a healthy weight, equalize your caloric intake and energy output.

If you are prone to gaining weight, the overeat-underexercise formula is most often the reason. But eating the amount of food your body needs to lose weight (translation: following a calorie-restricted, traditional diet) isn't working for the millions of Americans who diet, lose weight, and then gain it back . . . and more. Other parts of the scientific weight loss–weight gain puzzle include: the kinds of food you eat, whether your lifestyle includes regular physical activity, whether you turn to food to cope with stressful situations in your life, your genes and biology, and your age and health status.

With the Enlightened Diet, we are suggesting additional reasons for overeating and being overweight. Not only does the Enlightened Diet target known eating styles that influence how much you weigh, but it also reveals newly discovered biological, psychological, spiritual, and social reasons for your food choices and eating behaviors that determine whether you gain or lose weight. Indeed, our research on the seven eating styles reveals the key reason most of us fail to lose weight and keep it off is the fault of diets themselves. After all, they do not address the *underlying* and multidimensional causes of overeating and weight gain that comprise the Enlightened Diet.

To date, hundreds of research studies link weight, health, and wellness to what you eat (diet) and other lifestyle choices you make each day, such as exercise, stress management, and social support. Indeed, your diet and how you live are two of the most important, if not the most important, determinants of your physical, emotional, spiritual, and social well-being. Yet if you are overweight, or have been diagnosed with one or more of the myriad health problems that stem from obesity, from heart disease and diabetes to depression and social isolation, you've probably discovered that sound, supportive, scientifically based personal guidance that can lead to health and healing is sorely lacking.

We created the Enlightened Diet to help you identify obstacles keeping you from reaching your optimal weight, and we show you, step by step, how to overcome them. In this way, you are empowered to achieve your personal weight and wellness goals. Our program also reveals the food-related aspects of your lifestyle that cause—and cure— weight gain and associated illness. And, as you'll see, the weight loss skills, insights, and techniques you'll discover are personally tailored for you to do at your own pace, based on your personal needs.

The Seven Eating Styles

Are you a food fretter? A task snacker? An emotional eater? Or do you typically "flavor" food with all—or none—of the eating styles? The seven eating styles we discovered during our research on weight loss revealed new insights into why so many of us overeat and gain weight and what we can do about it. The eating styles are: food fretting, task snacking, emotional eating, fast foodism, solo dining, unappetizing atmosphere, and sensory disregard.[3] Throughout this book, we'll show you how to modify each eating style, so that it no longer leads to weight gain.

Here's how it works. The total eating style program in the book works by giving you the skills you need to fine-tune each of the eating styles, so that you can achieve and maintain your ideal weight. Fill out our personalized seven eating style profiles at the end of this chapter to find out which ones may be keeping you from staying slim. The quiz will reveal the degree to which you are practicing—or not—each eating style. In other words, you will discover how the *food choices* you most often make, and the *eating behaviors* you typically practice, work together to contribute to overeating and weight gain. Once you become aware of this, you will know the eating styles that need your attention the most, as well as those that may need minor modifications.

Once you discover your trouble spots and areas in which you can improve, each chapter gives you scientifically sound insights into the eating style, then a menu of choices and actions you can take that are the antidotes to overeating and weight gain. In other words, once you discover the eating styles that are holding you back, we give you an action plan that includes an abundance of personalized choices and options that you can practice and apply daily. These whole person nutrition and eating skills, tools, and insights are what you need to get slim and stay slim for life.

At the same time, you will be empowered to change the way you think about food, dieting, eating, and achieving and maintaining normal weight. The end result: the experience of whole person nutrition, wellness living, and weight loss.

In short, if there's a secret to successful dieting, the Enlightened Diet is it. With clearly defined and informed recommendations based on our research and other scientific studies, the Enlightened Diet provides a total resource for creating an individualized plan that's right for you. It accomplishes this by giving you the evidence-based insights you need to modify not only *what* you eat, but also how, why, when, with whom—even where.

Once you understand all aspects of your relationship to food and eating (biological, psychological, spiritual, and social), you will have a high level of awareness about what's leading you to overeat and gain weight. In turn, you can use these insights and wisdom to create conscious choices that optimize your relationship with food and eating. In other words, you discover how to turn a pattern of unsustainable food restriction into whole person nutrition and weight loss as a way of life. By "setting your table" this way, you will be empowered to create an action-oriented plan that turns overeating into optimal eating—in other words, to "diet" successfully for a lifetime.

We call our newly discovered patterns of overeating "styles" because they are a unique expression of the way you, personally, live or behave in relationship to food and food-related activities, from shopping and selecting food to eating food—even the atmosphere in which you dine. Think about the eating styles in the following way: every day you make a decision to style your hair in a manner that you believe is attractive, interesting, easy, and comfortable. Ultimately, your hairstyle reflects your taste and becomes typical of you; in other words, it becomes your personal style. When you're feeling good about your hair, you might say you're having a good hair day; when it's not looking its best, you may describe it as a bad hair day. And then there are days when your hairstyle is somewhere between looking either good or bad. As with good, bad, and in between hair days, each of the seven eating styles provides insights into the spectrum of your food-related behaviors. On one end of the continuum, you are eating optimally, while the other end reveals that you are more likely to overeat and gain weight.

What does it mean to eat optimally? It means you take the time to nourish your body with a balanced intake of nutrients (biological nutrition); you get pleasure from food so that you feel satisfied (psychological nutrition); you connect to the life force in food (spiritual nutrition); and, because we're social beings, you realize you thrive when you dine with others while sharing convivial conversation in pleasant surroundings (social nutrition).

These biological, psychological, spiritual, and social nutrition facets comprise the essence of our Whole Person Nutrition Model and Program, and the comprehensive food, eating, nutrition, and lifestyle plan in this book. The more you distance yourself from these multi-dimensional facets of food, the more you're likely to be practicing one or more of the seven overeating styles, which in turn, leads to increased risk for becoming overweight or obese.

We realize it may be tempting to skip through this part of the book and, instead, to fill out the personal eating style questionnaire ("What's Your Eating Style?"), then to turn immediately to the chapter that most fits your profile. Taking only the first step is a good way to start, but it isn't likely to get you the results you want. That's because reaping the relationship-to-food rewards of our program asks that you "be here now," that you begin to relate to food and eating as an "in the moment" experience, and that you start—and continue—the journey by familiarizing yourself with all elements of our Whole Person Nutrition Model and Program, so that you can master the program, starting now.

With this overview of the seven eating styles, you will discover how to restyle your food life by discovering how to eat in order to lose weight and at the same time to enjoy food and the experience of eating. Each chapter will give you the tools, skills, and guidelines you need to accomplish this. Right now, though, we want to first shed light on the seven eating styles we've discovered that lead to overeating and weight gain, most of which have been overlooked by dieters, health professionals, and the diet industry. As you'll see, each style decodes the many reasons so many of us overeat and gain weight, while at the same time, each eating style—indeed, this entire book—offers the solution to the cycle.

Food Fretting

Good food, bad food. Legal food, illegal food. Sinful food, pure food. The food fretting eating style is overly concerned about and focused on food, as well as projecting moral judgment onto what we and others *should* eat. If you are often filled with thoughts about what you or others should or shouldn't eat, traditional dieting, or the "right" way to eat, or you tend to measure your self-worth and that of others based on what or how much is eaten, the food fretting eating style is a key contributor to your overeating.

Do you see yourself in any of the following examples of food fretting?

"I was good today," you may think when you've managed to avoid unhealthful foods, stick to your diet, and eat what you think you should.

"When my food cravings become powerful and I eat foods that are bad, I feel so guilty," is typical self-think for many food fretters.

"She should resist that sinful chocolate cake. Doesn't she have any will power?" you might think as you watch a person eat what she "shouldn't."

Overcoming this eating style begins first with recognizing such judgmental, fret-filled chatter about food and eating. Being honest with yourself will be challenging, in part because being critical and feeling anxious about food has become common in our culture. The work you do to overcome this eating style is well worth the effort because it will enable you to replace fret-filled self-think with smart-think that will empower you to overcome this weight-promoting eating style.

In chapter 2, "Food Fretting," we'll reveal the pitfalls of the judgmental dimension of eating. For instance, as you'll see, a key underlying element of this weight-inducing eating style is traditional dieting, and then berating ourselves if we go off the diet. But the many food-fretting guidelines we provide for overcoming fret-filled thoughts and recriminating behaviors about food and food choices—for both yourself and others—show you how to identify food fretting, and then what you can do about it. In other words, we will give you the specific strategies you'll need to turn weight-inducing judgmental thoughts and activities into a whole-person, nonjudgmental eating style so that you may enjoy food in light of its being a social, ceremonial, sensual pleasure—that doesn't lead to weight gain.

Task Snacking

Some call it "multitasking"; the French call it "vagabond eating"; many others in America think it's "normal." However it's perceived, if you often eat meals or snacks while working by yourself in front of your computer, while driving, watching TV, or standing at the kitchen counter, shopping with a friend, or talking on the phone, it's likely that the "task snacking" eating style is increasing your odds of becoming overweight or obese.

With this eating style, you will discover how to rearrange your environment—both internally and externally. We will show you how to work when you work, drive when you drive, and eat when you eat, rather than eating while doing other activities. At the same time, you will find that making simple choices about eating mindfully can lead to big changes in overcoming overeating.

In chapter 3, "Task Snacking," you will discover the complex of related busyness behaviors and how they can contribute to weight gain. The antidote is offered later in the chapter, where you will learn how to break the cycle of merging eating with other activities. As you'll see, eliminating task snacking completely isn't necessarily the goal; instead, we'll give you easy-to-take actions you can do right now to cut down on your food-related multitasking and, in turn, reduce your overeating . . . and weight.

Emotional Eating

Most of us are familiar with the phrase "emotional eating," a term that refers to those who turn to comfort food to soothe negative feelings, such as depression, anxiety, or loneliness, but also to enhance joyous, positive, celebratory emotions in response to, let's say, a wedding, birthday, or promotion. If you often eat to manage your feelings and to self-soothe—in other words, for reasons other than hunger—it's likely you're an emotional eater. Some health professionals describe this eating style as "compulsive overeating" or "food addiction." No matter what it's called, many of us turn to food to relieve emotional tension because it works. After all, doesn't eating certain foods or even thinking about eating serve as a distraction from emotions that may be making you feel uncomfortable?

It may not come as a surprise to you that our research revealed that emotional eating is the strongest predictor of overeating and becoming overweight and obese and, therefore, the key contributor to weight gain. What *is* groundbreaking, though, are the specific emotions we've identified—the family of emotions—that are strongly linked with the likelihood you'll overeat. In chapter 4, "Emotional Eating," we will reveal the feelings that most strongly predict overeating. We'll also give you other insights into this overeating style, such as breakthrough brain-chemistry research, which reveals how turning to certain foods may mean you're self-medicating, which, in turn, may set off a binge in order to feel better. In chapter 4, we shed light on the foods—and specific nutrients in them—that can bust the blues, boost memory, cut carb cravings, and more; in essence, this chapter will give you the nutritional insights, skills, and tools you'll need to make feel-good food choices.

Fast Foodism

A donut or sugary cereal for breakfast; a McDonald's double-burger with fries for lunch; and a supersized pizza, perhaps placed casually onto the dining table in its cardboard box, for dinner—add several servings of soft drinks throughout the day, and you have a profile of the fast food cuisine that is typical for many Americans. Not surprisingly, this eating style is strongly linked with overeating, overweight, and obesity—and it threatens more than your waistline.

As you will discover, we qualify the fast foodism overeating style with the phrase "as often as possible," to ensure that you don't interpret this overeating style or its solution as more dietary dogma, or as more rules and regulations for you to follow. As with all elements of the Enlightened Diet, our intention is to help you think of what and how you eat as a spectrum rather than as an all-or-nothing, black-or-white dietary dogma.

To help you accomplish this, chapter 5, "Fast Foodism," will reveal foods linked with overeating and ensuing weight gain; we'll also show you what's in the foods that keeps you from achieving your weight and health goals, and how such a diet and eating style threatens more than your waistline. Then we will give you the solution to changing your relationship to this overeating style by demystifying optimal eating. To jump-start you, we will also give you a plethora of practical tips, exercises, and strategies, so you can choose the foods that will help you achieve and maintain an optimal relationship to food, vitality, health, and well-being for a lifetime.

Solo Dining

The overeating style in chapter 6, "Solo Dining," will show you how to turn dining with others into a balm for body, heart, and soul. As your eating style shifts from a "me" mentality to a "we" awareness—and, more and more, you share food and the dining experience with others—you'll be taking yet another step toward fulfillment and weight loss.

As extraordinarily simple as the overeating style of solo dining appears, beware: it is a two-edged sword in that it can be both easy and difficult to implement. As many of you know, the demands of home, family, and work can make it challenging to carve out time to dine with others. Yet, once you learn the amazing healing possibilities of this eating style, you'll instantly begin to reap the benefits. To help you do this, "Solo Dining" will reveal the complex of related dining-alone behaviors and how they can contribute to overeating, as well as the "ingredients" and skills you need to create and enjoy dining experiences with others. With this eating style, you'll have yet another insight to eat optimally and to succeed at enhancing your relationship with food and eating.

Unappetizing Atmosphere

You may find it amazing to consider that the atmosphere in which you eat may make a difference in whether you overeat and gain weight, but it does. The unappetizing atmosphere eating style is powerful in that, once you implement it, it will provide instant gratification because it will quickly improve the quality of your life by enhancing how you feel, both physically and emotionally; it may even improve your relationships—with others as well as with food.

With this eating style, you will focus on the psychological and physical dining aesthetics of your life—from the atmosphere in your home to your surroundings at the office, in restaurants, drive-through restaurants, or at the home of family and friends. If you intend to be successful at overcoming overeating over the long term, this eating style will serve as a reminder to strengthen your resolve.

Chapter 7, "Unappetizing Atmosphere," will reveal more about the often overlooked contribution that ambiance and your surroundings play in overeating and weight gain, while the "Rx" we offer will give you a rich repository of strategies for accessing the healing power inherent in a relaxing, delightful, aesthetically pleasing, and welcoming dining atmosphere. We'll also show you what constitutes a pleasant dining milieu, and how to create and choose one as often as possible.

Sensory Disregard

A sensory and spiritual relationship to food, eating, and the dining experience may be the most overlooked aspect of overeating and ensuing weight gain. The problem is that most of us don't even know what it means to relate to food in this way, let alone have a clue about how to turn it into a key whole person eating style. Be assured that we will demystify the sensory disregard eating style for you. As a matter of fact, of all the eating styles we've identified, sensory and spiritual eating has the largest number of food-related experiences that are linked with optimal eating and weight.

Be assured that with this eating style, we will not be suggesting that you meditate on your meals for hours each day. Rather, you will discover how implementing each of the elements of the spiritual and sensual eating style will turn your meals into a palate-pleasing adventure that nourishes both body and soul. At the same time, whether you're taking a tea break, sharing brunch with friends, or shopping for food, this groundbreaking, but age-old eating style may eliminate what isn't working for you, while turning your day-to-day dining experiences into a sensory experience that will lead to less overeating and optimal weight.

Consider this: even if this eating style is unfamiliar territory for you, it is still likely it is a major contributor to your overeating. If so, chapter 8, "Sensory Disregard," will give you insights into the price your mind, body, and waistline pay if you typically make meals and eat them without flavoring them with sensory and spiritual ingredients. Then we will empower you to experience food and dining as a symphonic masterpiece, for when you eat *from* the heart, you also reap the rewards of enjoying—indeed, savoring—your meals in a meaningful way.

Enlightened Exercise

After you discover the eating styles, our "Enlightened Exercise" perspective and menu of motion choices, in chapter 9, will give you insights into the benefits of including motion and movement (exercise) as a pivotal ingredient in living the Enlightened Diet. (Remember, the Enlightened Diet is a way of life, not a restrictive diet and exercise regimen.) This chapter includes a menu of movement options from which you may choose, based on your personal in-motion preferences, inclinations, and lifestyle. Finally, to demystify what the Enlightened Diet looks like in real life, chapter 10, "In Action," shows you how to practice each eating style each day.

Making Meals Memorable

When we ask people in our workshops to share a memorable meal or dining experience, without fail, the stories they share include all elements of the Enlightened Diet: (1) they anticipated the meal and ate it with pleasure, without judgment or anxiety; (2) they focused on the food and its flavor; (3) they enjoyed, indeed relished, the food, while filled with positive feelings; (4) the meal was made with fresh ingredients; (5) they shared the food and the dining experience with others; (6) they dined in pleasing surroundings; and (7) they appreciated the meal's sensory and spiritual ingredients. In other words, their meal memories instinctively included all elements of the Enlightened Diet: pleasure, mindfulness, feel-good feelings, fresh food, social ingredients, aesthetics awareness, and eating *from* the heart.

Whether the fare is simple or sublime, it's possible for you, too, to have memorable meals and to manage your weight at the same time. How? By practicing and living the seven eating styles in a whole person nutrition way. We'll show you how to begin with the following "What's Your Eating Style?" questionnaire we've created for you. By completing each section, tallying your scores, then interpreting your results, you'll discover your strengths as well as any weaknesses that are contributing to your overeating and weight gain and, therefore, the areas that need your attention.

By becoming familiar with the overeating styles that are currently integral to your life, you'll be able to take an active role in changing what isn't working for you. Step by step, we will give you practical, specific, action-filled whole person nutrition tools, skills, and strategies to make the changes that you, personally, need to be successful in creating an optimal, positive relationship to food and eating, and a healthy weight for a lifetime.

What's Your Eating Style?

Where are you now? We created your personal eating style profile, so you can find out how much—or how little—each eating style may be contributing to your overeating and weight gain. Consider the profile to be a lighthouse that helps you get your bearings, a guide for determining your eating style whereabouts so that you can choose the direction that will lead you to the destination of your dreams.

Once you have insights into your eating styles, you can use each chapter in *The Enlightened Diet* as a guide to unlocking the code to your overeating. Completing the profile prior to reading the book will also give you a baseline you can use over time to measure improvements and changes in each eating style.

Checking the checkpoints. After you check off the boxes and tally your total score, you will have a clearer perspective about the eating styles that are working for you, as well as a better understanding of areas you may want to improve. You'll also be taking the first step toward getting acquainted with each eating style, so you can benefit from them each time you eat.

Tallying your scores. To see where you are now, complete each eating style questionnaire below by checking the boxes that best represent your current eating style. As you fill out the profile, please note that some of the eating style questionnaires have two sections. For these eating styles, score the top section by tallying all plus (+) numbers; tally the bottom section by adding all the minus (-) numbers. Then, to get your eating style score, subtract the minus subtotal from the plus subtotal and enter the result on the total line at the bottom of each eating style profile.

Interpreting your scores. At the bottom of each style profile, you will also find a scoring key that tells you whether your score ranks as "excellent," "good," "satisfactory," or "needs improvement." To discover your total Eating Style Score for all seven eating styles, add the totals from each of the seven profiles; then read the interpretation about your Eating Style Score at the end of the profile.

Getting Started

Because all of the eating styles are interrelated, each has a powerful influence on whether you overeat and how much you weigh. The good news is that regardless of your starting point, if you change one eating style, it likely will lead to changes in others. Or you may decide to make more dramatic changes by implementing each element of the Enlightened Diet all at once. Or perhaps you may choose to make changes in your eating styles by targeting specific behaviors and choices within each eating style. There's no right or wrong way to follow the Enlightened Diet. Rather, use all the insights and strategies in each chapter to decide what will work best for you, personally.

Food Fretting Personal Profile

For each question, check the box in the column that best represents your "anxious eating" dynamic.

	Never	Rarely	Some-times	Usually	Almost Always	Always
	0	−1	−2	−3	−4	−5
1. I feel anxious about the best way to eat.	☐	☐	☐	☐	☐	☐
2. I feel good or righteous when I eat what I think I should.	☐	☐	☐	☐	☐	☐
3. When I overeat, I feel: bad	☐	☐	☐	☐	☐	☐
guilty	☐	☐	☐	☐	☐	☐
gluttonous	☐	☐	☐	☐	☐	☐
4. I judge others by what they eat.	☐	☐	☐	☐	☐	☐
5. I try different diets.	☐	☐	☐	☐	☐	☐
6. I count calories, fat grams, etc.	☐	☐	☐	☐	☐	☐
7. I obsess about food.	☐	☐	☐	☐	☐	☐
				Total Food Fretting Score: _____		

FOOD FRETTING SCORING KEY

0 to −7: Excellent   −15 to −21: Satisfactory
−8 to −14: Good   −22 or less: Needs improvement

Task Snacking Personal Profile

For each question, check the box in the column that best represents your task snacking dynamic.

	Never	Rarely	Some-times	Usually	Almost Always	Always
	0	−1	−2	−3	−4	−5
1. When I eat, I am:						
walking, rushing somewhere	❑	❑	❑	❑	❑	❑
at my desk at work	❑	❑	❑	❑	❑	❑
in my car	❑	❑	❑	❑	❑	❑
at my computer	❑	❑	❑	❑	❑	❑
talking on the phone	❑	❑	❑	❑	❑	❑
driving	❑	❑	❑	❑	❑	❑
watching tv	❑	❑	❑	❑	❑	❑
reading	❑	❑	❑	❑	❑	❑
	Total Task Snacking Score: _____					

TASK SNACKING SCORING KEY

0 to −8: Excellent   −15 to −19: Satisfactory

−9 to −14: Good   −20 or less: Needs improvement

Emotional Eating Personal Profile

For each question, check the box in the column that best represents your emotional eating dynamic.

	Never	Rarely	Some-times	Usually	Almost Always	Always
	0	+1	+2	+3	+4	+5
1. Before eating, I check my hunger level.	❑	❑	❑	❑	❑	❑
2. I eat only when I am hungry.	❑	❑	❑	❑	❑	❑
					Subtotal: + _____	

	Never	Rarely	Some-times	Usually	Almost Always	Always
	0	−1	−2	−3	−4	−5
3. I overeat.	❑	❑	❑	❑	❑	❑
4. After eating, I feel stuffed.	❑	❑	❑	❑	❑	❑
5. I have food cravings.	❑	❑	❑	❑	❑	❑
6. I eat because I feel: depressed	❑	❑	❑	❑	❑	❑
sad	❑	❑	❑	❑	❑	❑
anxious	❑	❑	❑	❑	❑	❑
angry	❑	❑	❑	❑	❑	❑
frustrated	❑	❑	❑	❑	❑	❑
happy	❑	❑	❑	❑	❑	❑
					Subtotal: − _____	
	Total Emotional Eating Score: (+) or (−) _____					

EMOTIONAL EATING SCORING KEY

10 to −1: Excellent   −13 to −23: Satisfactory
−2 to −12: Good   −24 or less: Needs improvement

Fast Foodism Personal Profile

For each question, check the box in the column that best represents your fast foodism dynamic.

	Never	Rarely	Some-times	Usually	Almost Always	Always
	0	+1	+2	+3	+4	+5
1. I eat fresh:						
fruits	❑	❑	❑	❑	❑	❑
vegetables	❑	❑	❑	❑	❑	❑
whole grains	❑	❑	❑	❑	❑	❑
legumes	❑	❑	❑	❑	❑	❑
nuts	❑	❑	❑	❑	❑	❑
seeds (e.g., sunflower, flax)	❑	❑	❑	❑	❑	❑
2. I eat meals that are homemade.	❑	❑	❑	❑	❑	❑

Subtotal: + _____

	Never	Rarely	Some-times	Usually	Almost Always	Always
	0	−1	−2	−3	−4	−5
3. I eat food that is:						
fast (such as McDonald's)	❑	❑	❑	❑	❑	❑
processed (canned, packaged)	❑	❑	❑	❑	❑	❑
prepared (deli, take-out)	❑	❑	❑	❑	❑	❑
sweet (donuts, muffins)	❑	❑	❑	❑	❑	❑
fried (potato chips, chicken)	❑	❑	❑	❑	❑	❑

Subtotal: − _____

Total Fast Foodism Score: (+) or (−) _____

FAST FOODISM SCORING KEY

35 to 23: Excellent   10 to −1: Satisfactory
22 to 11: Good   −2 or less: Needs improvement

Solo Dining Personal Profile

For each question, check the box in the column that best represents your solo dining dynamic.

	Never	Rarely	Some-times	Usually	Almost Always	Always
	0	+1	+2	+3	+4	+5
1. I eat with: friends family members	☐ ☐	☐ ☐	☐ ☐	☐ ☐	☐ ☐	☐ ☐
2. I eat at home at the dining table.	☐	☐	☐	☐	☐	☐
3. I enjoy preparing meals for friends.	☐	☐	☐	☐	☐	☐
4. I enjoy holiday feasts with others.	☐	☐	☐	☐	☐	☐
5. I celebrate special occasions with others with festive foods.	☐	☐	☐	☐	☐	☐
6. I prepare and share special meals for friends and family.	☐	☐	☐	☐	☐	☐
7. When eating alone, I often think about special people in my life, or memorable meals I've enjoyed with others.	☐	☐	☐	☐	☐	☐
					Subtotal: + _____	

	Never	Rarely	Some-times	Usually	Almost Always	Always
	0	−1	−2	−3	−4	−5
8. I eat alone.	☐	☐	☐	☐	☐	☐
9. I plan secret overeating sessions.	☐	☐	☐	☐	☐	☐
10. I dine with others, then afterward binge by myself.	☐	☐	☐	☐	☐	☐
11. I stand at the counter while eating.	☐	☐	☐	☐	☐	☐
					Subtotal: − _____	
				Total Solo Dining Score: (+) or (−) _____		

SOLO DINING SCORING KEY

40 to 28: Excellent   15 to 4: Satisfactory
27 to 16: Good   3 or less: Needs improvement

Unappetizing Atmosphere Personal Profile

For each question, check the box in the column that best represents your unappetizing atmosphere dynamic.

	Never	Rarely	Some-times	Usually	Almost Always	Always
	0	+1	+2	+3	+4	+5
1. The atmosphere in which I prepare and eat food is:						
serene	❏	❏	❏	❏	❏	❏
pleasing	❏	❏	❏	❏	❏	❏
fun	❏	❏	❏	❏	❏	❏
2. After eating, I feel:						
relaxed	❏	❏	❏	❏	❏	❏
calm	❏	❏	❏	❏	❏	❏
alert	❏	❏	❏	❏	❏	❏
					Subtotal: + _____	

	Never	Rarely	Some-times	Usually	Almost Always	Always
	0	–1	–2	–3	–4	–5
3. The atmosphere in which I prepare and eat food is:						
hectic	❏	❏	❏	❏	❏	❏
tense	❏	❏	❏	❏	❏	❏
					Subtotal: – _____	
		Total Unappetizing Atmosphere Score: (+) or (–) _____				

UNAPPETIZING ATMOSPHERE SCORING KEY

30 to 22: Excellent   13 to 6: Satisfactory
21 to 14: Good   5 or less: Needs improvement

Sensory Disregard Personal Profile

For each question, check the box in the column that best represents your sensory disregard dynamic.

	Never	Rarely	Some-times	Usually	Almost Always	Always
	0	+1	+2	+3	+4	+5
1. I plan and prepare meals: with care	❑	❑	❑	❑	❑	❑
with appreciation	❑	❑	❑	❑	❑	❑
2. While dining, I consider my surroundings.	❑	❑	❑	❑	❑	❑
3. I express gratitude for food through prayer, blessings, heartfelt thankfulness.	❑	❑	❑	❑	❑	❑
4. I honor the mystery of life in food.	❑	❑	❑	❑	❑	❑
5. Before and during eating, I focus on the food's: color	❑	❑	❑	❑	❑	❑
aroma	❑	❑	❑	❑	❑	❑
portion size	❑	❑	❑	❑	❑	❑
flavors	❑	❑	❑	❑	❑	❑
6. I "eat" with my senses, by: appreciating the presentation	❑	❑	❑	❑	❑	❑
tasting textures	❑	❑	❑	❑	❑	❑
savoring scents	❑	❑	❑	❑	❑	❑
7. I focus solely on food and the experience of dining.	❑	❑	❑	❑	❑	❑
8. I appreciate the web of humanity (farmers, grocers) surrounding food.	❑	❑	❑	❑	❑	❑
9. I consider the elements of nature that create food.	❑	❑	❑	❑	❑	❑
10. I eat with loving regard for food.	❑	❑	❑	❑	❑	❑
11. After eating, I: savor the moment	❑	❑	❑	❑	❑	❑
reflect on the meal	❑	❑	❑	❑	❑	❑
Total Sensory Disregard Score: _____						

SENSORY DISREGARD SCORING KEY

72 to 90: Excellent   54 to 71: Good
53 to 36: Satisfactory   35 or less: Needs improvement

Your Eating Style Score

To find your Total Whole Person Nutrition Eating Style Score:

1. Enter the **positive** scores from each of the seven eating styles in the "Positive Subtotals" column.
2. Enter the **negative** scores from each of the seven eating styles in the "Negative Subtotals" column.
3. For your "Total Whole Person Nutrition Eating Style Score," subtract the total negative subtotals from the total positive subtotals.

Eating Style	Positive Subtotals	Negative Subtotals
Food Fretting	_____	_____
Task Snacking	_____	_____
Emotional Eating	_____	_____
Fast Foodism	_____	_____
Solo Dining	_____	_____
Unappetizing Atmosphere	_____	_____
Sensory Disregard	_____	_____

Positive Total: _____   **Negative Total:** _____

Total Whole Person Nutrition Eating Style Score: _____

Evaluating Your Score

131 or more: Excellent. Congratulations! The "excellent" level is comparable to an A+. Your relationship with food is mostly satisfying and gratifying. In other words, you eat less and enjoy it more most of the time. Both what and how you eat is beneficial to your weight, your overall health, and your quality of life.

A score of "excellent" suggests that you are already practicing many of the elements of the Enlightened Diet. To reap even more benefits, look over your answers for each eating style, then target even more changes you could make that would lead to even more delightful dining. Then turn to the chapters on each eating style for more insights and tips on eating even more optimally.

130 to 55: Good. You're doing fairly well! The "good" level falls between the grades of A and B+. The foods you choose, how you eat, and with whom you eat are typically positive and beneficial. You eat optimally sometimes; when you're not able to—or choose not to—you let it go.

To reap even more benefits, look over your answers for each eating style, and decide whether there are changes you would like to make that would bring you closer to the Enlightened Diet. Then turn to the chapters on each eating style—particularly those to which you seem to have some resistance—for more insights and tips on eating even more optimally.

54 to −24: Satisfactory. Food and eating are often issues for you. If you ranked "satisfactory," the way you typically eat is comparable to between a grade of B and C. You may have some confusion about what and how to eat optimally, or your eating style hasn't been a priority for you so far. Your relationship to food and eating are fairly typical, which leaves lots of room for making beneficial changes.

A score of "satisfactory" suggests that you may be finding it challenging to practice many of the elements of the Enlightened Diet. To reap more benefits, look over your answers for each eating style to target specific changes you would like to make that would lead you closer to the Enlightened Diet. Then turn to the chapters on each eating style for more insights and tips on eating even more optimally.

−25 or less: Needs improvement. Your overall eating style is far from optimal. Decide whether you want to take steps toward improving your relationship with food. To help you do this, first read the "Stages of Change" section in chapter 2, "Food Fretting." Once you're clear about wanting to make changes, get some ideas for how to begin by retaking the "What's Your Eating Style?" questionnaire, or look over the questions in each section of the questionnaire for some quick and easy ways to implement ideas and suggestions.

A score of "needs improvement" suggests that you would benefit a lot by learning about, and then living, all the elements of the Enlightened Diet. To get started, look over your answers for each eating style to target specific changes you would like to make that will bring you closer to living the Enlightened Diet. Remember, small steps can lead to big benefits. Then turn to the chapters on each eating style for more insights and tips on eating even more optimally.

Chapter 2

Food Fretting

$\text{R}\!\!\!\!\text{x}$: Perceive food and the experience of eating as a social, ceremonial, sensual pleasure.

Not long ago, as I chatted with a friend in front of my local supermarket while enjoying a piece of delicious dark chocolate, an acquaintance from our local health club walked by. "I see you," she said in response to my munching on what she perceived to be forbidden food. Knowing that I'm knowledgeable about nutrition, this same health club contact often approached me as I worked out to solicit my opinion about what and how much she should eat to lose weight. Other times, she would walk up to me, and right after "Hello, Deborah" she would give me a detailed report on what she had had for breakfast, lunch, and dinner the previous day, based on the diet du jour she was following. "What do you think of this diet?" she would ask.

This same woman would occasionally take the liberty of telling me about a meal she had eaten at a favorite restaurant. Did she make a "good" choice? Or not? And then there were the confessions about "sinful" desserts or "bad" carbs. She knew she "shouldn't eat these foods," but she missed them when she was "on a diet," so much so that she would often scarf down too much too quickly. "I know. I've completely blown my diet," would be her self-recriminating, guilt-laden lament. Then she would vow to "get back on track tomorrow."

My health club acquaintance is a textbook example of food fretting in action: dieting as a way of life; guilt, anxiety, and righteousness about the "best" way to eat; noticing what someone is eating, then judging it, even commenting on it; judging one's own food choices; eating by number (such as calorie counting and weight watching); and obsessing about food.

Although dieting, a judgmental attitude, and anxiety about food may seem as if they don't have much in common, they share the distinguishing characteristics of a food fretter: apprehension about what food to eat; feeling gluttonous when eating foods you think you shouldn't; guilt when you go off your diet; and comparing yourself with others and then judging the differences. The key characteristic, though, is obsessing about food.

If you're a food fretter, you may also experience an alternating sense of righteousness or self-disdain—depending on how you're doing on your diet on a particular day. You tend to regard food with anxiety, and to judge what and how you eat as "good" or "bad" behaviors. You may even feel inadequate or envious when you see a thin person. The end result: you fill much of your day-to-day thinking and ruminating about food, "eating right," being thin—and often overeating.

Dieting Doldrums

If you think the food fretter's relationship to food, eating, dieting, and weight loss is normal—you're right. In America, 83 percent of college women diet no matter how much they weigh; two-thirds of Americans have tried some kind of weight loss diet; almost 50 percent of women are dieting on any given day, as is one in four men; and almost half of ten-year-old girls feel better about themselves when they're dieting.[1]

Clearly, dieting is a national obsession that is evident in the over forty billion dollars we spend each year on dieting and related products. Yet as our fixation on dieting increases, so, too, do our waistlines.

More than 65 percent of adults over twenty-five are either overweight or obese, up from 58 percent in 1983. And one in five children is expected to be obese (a BMI equal to 30 or more) by 2010.[2]

Regardless, millions of concerned Americans turn for help to diet books, surgery, or expensive spas; still other gullible and desperate dieters succumb to quick-fix claims such as "Eat all you want and still lose weight" or "Melt away fat while you sleep." All the while they remain oblivious to the secrets of successful dieting: first and foremost, stop dieting.

Meet EDNOS

What's key to understanding the futility of food fretting and its family member, dieting, is that although it is "normal," it doesn't translate into weight loss: more than 95 percent of dieters regain their lost weight in one to five years. Just as disheartening, 35 percent of "normal" dieters progress to pathological, obsessive dieting, while others develop full-blown eating disorders (EDs), such as anorexia nervosa, bulimia nervosa, or binge eating disorder (BED), serious psychological conditions. What they have in common is that the sufferer is obsessed with food, diet, and often body image, which puts both quality of life and health at extreme risk.

Meet EDNOS, the acronym for an "Eating Disorder Not Otherwise Specified." This term covers that gray area of disordered eating patterns that lies between optimal, healthful eating and clinical eating disorders. For instance, people with an EDNOS may diet chronically, focus on weight constantly, or binge occasionally. In other words, food and eating are a major source of stress for people with EDNOS. And this means they are food fretters and at risk for overeating and weight gain.

I remember as a child watching my mother jump into the dieting ditch. She and a few of her friends had just returned from their first Weight Watchers meeting, in the early days of Weight Watchers, when its founder, Jean Neidich, was at the helm, and being a member meant weighing your serving sizes and yourself. Sitting at our kitchen table, I watched in amazement as my mother and her friends displayed the little tabletop food scales they would use to weigh their food. On the surface, the dieting ritual they had just learned and were practicing with food from the fridge seemed like harmless fun and an opportunity to socialize. But now, when I revisit the scene from the perspective of an adult and researcher who now knows about food obsession and dieting, I perceive that evening as the start of my mother's formalized, ritualized food fretting. She told me that as a young adult, she often tried to will herself to abstain from foods she enjoyed so that she could "keep her figure"; now, as an adult and the mother of two children, watching her weight by dieting, weighing, and counting had become a way of life.

My mother's experience is typical of dieters: she entered the world of food fretting gradually, with high expectations of success—losing weight and maintaining a healthy weight. But because she didn't know that she was pursuing a seemingly simple, seemingly achievable vision that was really radical and difficult, she struggled with the battle of the bulge for years.

Scientific Insights into the Dieting Dilemma

Recent scientific discoveries that were not available to my mother's generation have a lot to tell us today about why dieting and obsessing about food doesn't work—and what you can do to escape, permanently, from the dieting gulag in which many of us are confined.

When we discovered the seven eating styles that form the Enlightened Diet, we realized that losing weight and keeping it off is based on a complex matrix of food- and eating-based thoughts, behaviors, and feelings. The results you want—enjoying food and eating as a way of life that leads naturally to weight loss and physical health, emotional well-being, spiritual sustenance, and social support—may call for making long-term changes not only to what you eat and how much you eat, but especially to why and how you eat.

As a first step toward getting from where you are to where you want to be, consider three key questions that lie at the heart of getting off the food fretting treadmill of dieting and obsessing about food. Are your weight goals and expectations realistic? Is there a "best" (regimented) diet that works long term? Are you really ready to make the changes necessary to lose weight, or do you just think (and hope) you are?

Reframing Successful Dieting

A close look at most diet and weight loss programs reveals that they ask you to set a "goal weight," the number of pounds you want to lose to achieve a targeted weight. If you buy into this popular norm, you may be setting yourself up for failure. Consider novel research on goal weight and how it sabotages success, conducted by obesity researcher Gary D. Foster in the late 1990s. Foster, who is director for the Center for Weight and Eating Disorders at Temple University, wanted to explore why so many of us give up and fail at dieting. To find out, he and his team asked sixty obese women to identify how many pounds they would need to lose to achieve what they consider their ideal "dream" weight, "happy" weight, "acceptable" weight, and "disappointed" weight. At the end of the forty-eight-week weight loss program, almost half didn't achieve even their disappointed weight. When the researchers replicated the study with 154 overweight people, including men, again those least successful at losing weight were the most obese with the most unrealistic weight loss "dream" goals.[3]

If we didn't know that obsessing about weight contributes to failure, we might think that the dieters didn't have the willpower to reach their goal weight. We might imagine that the diet they followed was too hard and strict, that the dieters weren't really committed to losing weight, or perhaps that there was a biological or genetic reason for their failure. But the food fretting mentality inherent in targeting a goal weight suggests something quite different. It tells us that obsessing about a particular number (how much you would like to weigh) isn't an effective or realistic (or pleasant) way to lose weight. It simply doesn't work. And not only doesn't it work, but with such high dropout rates, there also seems to be something that's actually counterproductive to dropping pounds when you set a goal weight.

A more recent, comprehensive national study led by principal investigator Riccardo Dalle Grave, an obesity researcher from Italy, supports Foster's findings and the futility of food fretting as an effective way to lose weight. When Dalle Grave and his colleagues assessed the weight loss expectations of 1,785 obese people seeking treatment in twenty-three medical centers, they discovered that dropouts had more pounds to lose to achieve their "dream" weight compared with the continuers who finished the study. Indeed, the strongest predictor that people would drop out of the study was the degree to which their weight loss expectations were unrealistic.[4]

Both Foster and Dalle Grave interpreted their goal weight studies in a similar way: because unrealistic weight loss expectations increase the likelihood that an overweight person will give up and drop out, more modest weight loss goals may be a more realistic way to lose weight. But stopping food fretting and reframing what constitutes successful weight loss has even larger implications: even modest weight loss can bring big health benefits.

There are three interesting insights we can learn from these studies. The first is that unrealistic expectations and goals about weight loss lead to disappointment and giving up. And feeling that your efforts to lose weight are futile is a clear predictor that you will, indeed, go off your diet and fail to lose weight. The second interesting insight is that the goal weights chosen by the obese participants in the studies were three times as great as their actual weight lost. The message we can take away from this is that you would be wise to reduce your initial goal, perhaps by as much as two-thirds, then set another modest goal weight after your initial weight loss phase. Another key insight addresses how you think of yourself. Since participants' body image and self-esteem were tied to how much weight they wanted to lose (the lower the self-image, the more extreme and unrealistic the goal weight), you would be smart to reverse the formula: work on esteem and body image to reduce unrealistic expectations and increase your likelihood of success.

If you suffer from one or more medical problems related directly to your weight, knowing the big benefits you can achieve with just a small amount of weight loss is powerful news. Lose just ten pounds and your triglyceride levels (a risk factor for heart disease) can drop as much as 34 percent, your total cholesterol can decrease 16 percent, LDL (bad) cholesterol can decrease 12 percent, and HDL (good) cholesterol can increase 18 percent. If you have high blood pressure or diabetes, you may be able to reduce or discontinue medications if you lose only 5 to 10 percent of your current weight. And if degenerative joint disease, such as osteoarthritis, is a problem for you, for every 2.2 pounds you lose, you reduce the stress on each knee by approximately five pounds per square inch. This weight loss could translate into delaying or negating the need for knee surgery.[5]

The message is clear: small changes can bring big benefits. Even modest but sustained weight loss, without targeting an ideal body weight, can improve many weight-related ailments and your overall health and well-being. And you're also likely to look better and to feel better about yourself.

As simple as it sounds, shifting your thinking from reaching an ideal weight to establishing reasonable expectations is a dramatic paradigm shift, according to Foster. In other words, reframing weight loss success calls for a major change in the diet-think that permeates our culture. But the health rewards of losing even a modest amount of weight are well worth the effort. And there's more good news: when you stop dieting and reframe your idea of successful weight loss, you'll also experience less stress around food, eating, and your weight, and more peace of mind.

Unrealistic weight loss goals may be a key food fretting culprit that keeps you from attempting to lose, or actually losing, weight and feeling good about yourself. But if changing the way you think about weight loss success is a key piece to the weight loss puzzle, would it be helpful if you also changed the way you think about diets themselves—especially if you knew that they not only hinder but also sabotage and destroy the likelihood that you'll lose weight and keep it off?

Diet More, Weigh More

The strongest food fretting predictor that you'll overeat and gain weight is traditional dieting. If you live your life on a diet and restrict your calories with the intention of losing weight, you're following a recipe not only for failure, but also for inverse results: you're actually putting yourself at risk to gain weight.

Earlier in this chapter, I mentioned that about 95 percent of those who lose weight on a traditional diet gain that weight back. If you've followed this track, it's likely you lost some weight while you were on the diet; after all, if you restrict your calories you will lose weight. But you're also likely to lose a lot more: muscle mass and a speedy metabolism; this is of special concern because if your muscles and your metabolism (the rate at which your body processes food) are in good shape, it'll be easier for you to lose weight and keep it off. But cut calories and your muscles and your metabolism weaken, sabotaging your weight loss. Here's why.

Muscles. The amount of energy (calories from food) your body needs each day is based on your basal metabolic rate, as well as your daily physical activity. For most or us, this equals 1,500 to 2,500 calories per day. Reduce your daily caloric intake to below what your body needs (in other words, go on a diet), to, say, 1,200 calories, and your body goes into survival mode. After all, it doesn't know you're a woman on a calorie-restricted diet whose goal is to fit into a size 6; no, your body thinks it's starving. To keep this from happening—especially if you are not exercising or doing weight resistant exercises—it turns to your muscle tissue and breaks it down for energy. And once you lose muscle mass, your body will need even fewer calories than it did prior to dieting; in other words, you'll need to consume even less food to lose weight or keep it off.

There's more bad news. Because your muscle mass is providing the energy you need, even if you lose maybe twenty-five pounds on your low-calorie diet, you'll lose both muscle and fat in equal amounts. *And your body will actually become more efficient at storing fat by slowing down your metabolism.*

Metabolism. When your metabolism is performing optimally, your body efficiently burns the calories from your food. If you don't eat enough food, though, your metabolism slows down and you don't burn calories as quickly. As you continue to starve yourself (at least, this is what your body thinks you're doing), your metabolism burns calories in food more slowly. When you stop your restrictive diet, your metabolism stays slow, making it easier for you to gain the weight back even faster, even if you still cut calories and eat less than before you decided to diet.

The bottom line: low-calorie diets make your body more efficient at storing fat—not losing it—and they slow down your metabolism, making it harder—not easier—for you to lose weight.

There's another catch-22 to cutting calories: you actually train your mind to obsess about food. Here's how it works. First, you're told to, or you decide to, visualize or imagine how you want to look at your "ideal" weight; some diet experts even suggest that you put a picture of a person at your "perfect" visualized weight on your refrigerator, so that it can serve as a reminder for you to stay on your diet each day. Then there are the food lists, exchanges, and points. Is this food permitted? Or not? Is it low carb or high fat? Whichever way you turn the grocery cart, it's geared toward your thinking and thinking and thinking about food—in other words, obsessing about it. Add this to the fact that you're being told to restrict what and how much you can't and shouldn't eat, and you're setting yourself up for a food mutiny! Ergo, you break your diet and eat the foods you've been craving—and as much of them as you allow your craving to drive you to eat.

The Four Diets Study

A recent research project that verifies diets are not the path to take for losing weight was motivated by the scarcity of studies on the topic. To find out whether popular diets (Atkins, Zone, Weight Watchers, and Ornish) work, whether there is a "best" diet that health practitioners can recommend to patients for weight loss and reduced risk of heart disease, researchers randomly assigned 160 overweight or obese adults aged twenty-two to seventy-two to one of the four wildly popular diets. During the first two months, both a doctor and a dietitian trained participants; then they were on their own for ten more months, until the weigh-in after a year of dieting.

When the results were tallied, the researchers discovered that while each diet significantly lowered bad cholesterol and increased good cholesterol, the dropout rate was substantial for all four diets: 53 percent for Atkins, 50 percent for Ornish, and 35 percent for Zone and Weight Watchers. And even though there was a slight average weight loss (4.6 to 7.3 pounds) after one year for those who managed to stay on one of the diets in the study, the number of pounds that were lost was so slight they didn't register as being statistically significant. The bottom line: no diet was better than another for weight loss; indeed, no study participants lost significant amounts of weight— regardless of the diet.

When I lecture about whole person nutrition and the seven eating styles, the question I'm asked most frequently is about the diet du jour. Many want to know which diet is best: Is it the Zone? *Eat Right 4 Your Type*? What do I think about Ornish (high carbohydrate/low fat) versus Atkins (high protein/high fat)? Which do I choose? The simple answer is that I don't choose because I know that diets don't work and that, instead, they lead to a sense of failure and self-esteem problems. Clearly, we're asking the wrong question (What's the best diet?), so we're getting the disappointing answer of ongoing weight gain; this may seem obvious, but it isn't. "I would suspect that most of the popular diet books in the bookstore are likely to produce weight loss if you follow the plan closely, since almost all plans are similar to the diets we studied, or to a cross between two of them," Michael L. Dansinger, MD, leader of the study, told WebMD. Dansinger continues: "Date the diets until you can find a life partner. The best way is to try a number of them . . ."[6]

What's accurate about Dansinger's suggestion is this: all weight loss diets work if dieters stick with them, but most don't for the reasons reviewed throughout this food fretting chapter. The four diets study confirms that all diets are challenging to stay with even with quality supervision (doctors and dietitians) and that for most people diets are not the answer for long-term weight loss.

Two other aspects of the study also caught our attention. First, we find it interesting that the Atkins, Zone, Weight Watchers, and Ornish diets that were chosen for the study have a lot in common: as with all diets, they omit the junk food and fast food that typically contribute to weight gain. What you are *not* eating plays a key role in whether you lose weight and keep it off. The other aspect of the study we find intriguing is its focus on each diet's proportion of macronutrients (carbohydrates, fat, and protein) and, to a lesser degree, micronutrients (such as vitamins and minerals); this is because the nutrient composition of food plays a key role in preventing, managing, or reversing a health condition, such as heart disease, diabetes, and depression. For instance, if you have heart disease or high cholesterol levels, the nutrient composition of the Ornish diet is optimal for reversal. But a diet's macro- and micronutrient balance isn't the key to optimizing the odds of weight loss success; balancing energy input (food) and output (physical activity) is.

Are You Really Ready to Lose Weight (or Do You Just *Want* To)?

Two decades ago, psychologists James Prochaska and Carlo DiClemente developed a model about how people change their lifestyle habits that was exceptional in three key ways. First, their model is supported by scientific studies. The second reason their ideas are unique is that they reframe successful lifestyle change that "sticks" as a step-by-step process, one that requires an experiential shift in a person's attitude, perception, and way of being. Without graduating through successive steps (five stages of change), individuals are more likely to fail to make lasting change. The third key component of their model tells us that as well as being a process, making long-term changes often involves setbacks, but with repeated efforts chances for success increase. In other words, change—such as losing weight—is not a black or white, all or nothing decision. Prochaska and DiClemente posit that to achieve lasting change, it's quite normal for people to make more than one attempt.[7]

Today, the psychologists' model is a cornerstone of a Transtheoretical Model of Change that is used by many health professionals and in dozens of behavior change programs that help people with behavioral addictions, such as gambling and workaholism, as well as substance abuse and addictions to drugs, cigarettes, and alcohol.

Although overeating and related disorders, such as binge eating disorder (BED), may feel like an addiction to those who struggle with their relationship to food, they technically aren't classed as addictions, because the chemical process linked to addictive behavior is different from the chemical changes in your brain that occur when you eat different foods (more about food and how it affects your mood in chapter 4, "Emotional Eating"). Rather, the food you eat may be considered a "substance" that creates chemical changes in your brain, which in turn influence your feelings. Those with EDNOS, who abuse food (and their bodies), are more likely to have a substance abuse problem, not an addiction. Another aspect of eating that makes what you eat and how you eat it different from a full-blown addiction is that food-related behaviors are considered to be deeply instilled habits that, for most of us, are hard to change—unless you find out where you are in the stages of change model, and then progress through each stage.

Stages of Change

The discovery of the stages of change gives us insights about how to change and specific strategies about how you can best help yourself in your effort to become a "successful loser."

The mistake most of us make when we think of losing weight by "going on a diet" is our ignorance of where we are in the stages of change cycle; this is because once you know which stage you're in, you can rationally and thoughtfully progress to the next stage. By not jumping ahead to a stage for which you may not be ready (such as dieting), you lower the odds of slipping back into old eating habits.

When Prochaska and DiClemente did their initial study, and they identified the five stages of change, it was with 872 people who were hoping to change their smoking habits. The five stages they discovered include: precontemplation, contemplation, preparation, action, and maintenance; the relapse stage refers to people who revert to precontemplation, contemplation, or preparation regarding their efforts to change.

The stages of change gives you powerful strategies that are specific to each stage. Take the time to identify the stage you're in, right now, and keep what you learn in mind as you gain knowledge about, and become skilled at, overcoming food fretting and the other eating styles in this book.

Precontemplation. This stage is a kind of precursor to the four other more formal stages that empower you to change your food choices, eating behaviors, and weight. If you're not interested in changing your food and eating habits ("This is the way I am; I'm big-boned."), if you're not concerned about being overweight ("Most Americans are overweight; I fit right in."), if you don't recognize you have a problem with food or weight ("It's society's problem, not mine."), you're in the precontemplation stage. You may also be ignorant of health risks linked with overweight or obesity and, instead, blame your weight on biology, metabolism, or genes you inherited from your parents. You're not too open to advice, and you're not yet contemplating change.

Contemplation. If you're thinking about changing what and how you eat, and you're kind of easing into it—perhaps you'll get to it tomorrow or sometime within the next few months—you are in the contemplation stage. At this stage, you may have some ambivalence, though, because considering a change in lifelong food habits can be a life-changing decision. As you progress through contemplation, you will come to a decision about your next step.

Preparation. If you're in this stage, you have decided to make a change; you have shifted from "I ought to" to "I'm going to." Making changes in your food choices and eating styles is just around the corner; you plan to do it within the next month. To prepare for success when you make your shift into action, you first weigh the pros and cons. What's the downside to what and how you're currently eating? What are the benefits you'll receive by changing your relationship to food? What's working well for you? What exactly needs to change? In other words, you're getting in touch with the downside of food fretting; at the same time, you are considering, organizing, and planning the benefits of de–food fretting. After you've considered the pros and cons, it is time to create your plan of action.

Action. During the preparation stage, you identified obstacles to making changes, as well as strengths you bring with you along the journey. You have entered the action stage when you have prepared yourself for change and have created specific steps. Now you're motivated and ready to implement the plan of action you've been thinking about for the past weeks or months. Not only are you clear about what you want to achieve, and how you're going to go about it, but you're also doing it and being it.

Maintenance. To maintain optimal food choices, eating behaviors, and weight loss calls for progressing through the above-mentioned stages until they become habitual. Keep in mind that it typically takes weeks (twelve weeks is a guesstimate) to change a habit, and to achieve lasting change. To increase the odds of success, this may be a good stage to weigh the benefits and obstacles you identified in the preparation stage, and make changes accordingly.

Relapse. The stages of change are not an all or none proposition (as are most diets); rather, they're a *process* of change, guidelines for transitioning from food fretting and yo-yo dieting to lasting change. Realize that it's common for many people to return to what is familiar and comfortable, even though it may not be what you want or what is good for you. Realize that many of us will relapse and return to prior eating habits and food choices for either a short or long time. This is not the time to get discouraged and give up. Rather, go back over the stages and plan how to overcome the obstacle that got in your way; when you have done this, return to the action stage. Be compassionate with yourself, then repeat each of the stages until the action stage becomes second nature.[8]

Are you really ready to lose weight, or do you just want to? Spend time with the stages and you'll know the answer. You'll know if and when you are really, really ready to change your food fretting when you understand the stage you're in, and you stay with that stage until you're truly ready, deep-down ready, to move to the contemplation stage or the action stage. Empowered by these self-insights, you'll be poised to turn the defeatism of traditional dieting upside down.

De–Food Fretting Strategies

There's a lot more you can do to de–food fret and overcome your food-related anxieties, obsessing, self-recrimination, judgment, and guilt. Here is a close look at what it takes to transcend food fretting and its cycle of dieting, anxiety, and obsessing about food and weight.

Don't diet. More and more research is linking traditional dieting with increased risk of weight gain. Consider *dieting* in the best sense of the word. The word *diet* comes from the Old French *diete* or Greek *diaeta*, which means "mode of life." Hippocrates, the father of modern medicine, used *diet* as a "prescribed mode of life," which eventually evolved into meaning "prescribed regime of food." We're suggesting that you *diet* as an expression of the ancient meaning of the word, as a way of life: you relate to eating as a social, ceremonial, and sensual delight, and to food as a gift that enhances your physical, emotional, spiritual, and social well-being.

Stop counting calories. Traditional diets that ask you to restrict calories and to eat-by-number (count calories, figure fat grams, etc.) to lose weight are no longer appropriate. To lose weight, you don't need more numbers; you need other ways of relating to food so that each time you eat you have an enjoyable experience that nourishes your entire being. Instead of staying lost in a maze of measurements, nutrients, and numbers, focus on fresh foods, their flavors, the profound pleasure of eating, and the delight you take in dining with others.

Halt judgment. In 1987, my father died abruptly of a heart attack; my mother also died of heart disease—congestive heart failure. Having worked as the nutrition educator with pioneering physician Dean Ornish on his first clinical trial for reversing heart disease and later as the director of nutrition in Europe on a similar research project, I knew a lot about nutrition, lifestyle, and health. Yet I still could not seem to find the "right" or "best" way to help my parents. I knew my parents understood the heart-healthy dietary information I'd given them, but in retrospect, I realize that the underlying message I was giving was, "You *should* be eating differently. You *should* stop eating familiar and comfortable foods. You *should* assess and analyze what you're eating." Should. It simply doesn't work—for you or others. How did I and so many of us learn to judge both ourselves and others' food choices and eating habits? I discovered that in the late 1800s, Puritan values still predominated in America, which meant that food was often perceived as sinful, or as good and bad; in other words, we projected moral values onto food—and still do. Instead, view food, eating, and the experience of dining as a celebration of life.

Give up guilt-tripping. Guilt and its relatives—self-reproach, shame, remorse, and blame—are part of a food fretter's relationship to food. It's all about what is "right" and what is "wrong." Eat something "wrong" that isn't on your diet, that you "shouldn't," that tastes "sinful," and, if you're a food fretter, you're likely to respond with guilt. The dictionary tells us that to feel guilty is to feel remorse about having done something wrong. That wrongdoing is linked with guilt has roots in the word's original meaning, derived from Old English, when it meant "crime."[9] Is eating food you "shouldn't" eat a crime? Or, as with the food fretter feeling of judgment, when you feel guilt over something you ate (or want to eat), are you projecting a moral value onto the food, and in the process making yourself miserable? Consider this: guilt isn't a real feeling. At its core lies the belief you've done something wrong, and now you must suffer for it. To break that conviction and get the upper hand over guilt, change what you choose to believe. Replace guilt-laden thoughts with a positive picture. Realize that you can't undo what was done, and . . . simply accept it. Finally, forgive yourself, for forgiveness is a necessity in any relationship—including the one you have with food.

Cease obsessing. If you're fixated on, and preoccupied with, food-related thoughts, feelings, and behaviors, if you think or worry about food or weight constantly and compulsively, you are obsessing. The way out is to step from the shade you're living in, into the sunshine. Meditation can help you do this.

Meditation and Meals

During a conversation in a café with a new acquaintance, I first realized the power of meditation as a path that leads to letting go of food fretting and replacing it with naturally occurring weight loss. Midway through our get-together, she told me she had lost twenty pounds as a side effect of meditating regularly. Accessing the wisdom within yourself through regular meditation is one path you can take to de–food fret and to create a more balanced relationship to food, eating, and your weight.

Meditation, and its myriad variations, has been a spiritual discipline espoused by world religions, philosophies, and traditions for thousands of years. In the East, yogis say it leads to a superconscious state that emerges from the cessation of thought; Taoists tell us it leads to a sense of harmony with all things and moments and a return to the depths of the self; while proponents of Zen perceive meditation as a path to sudden illumination. In the West, it is often linked with the mystical and monastic. The Kabbalah, Judaism's mystical teaching, turns to it to carry consciousness through various "gateways"; early Christian monks and saints used it as a stringent contemplative process to achieve spiritual exaltation; and Islam's spiritual Sufis interpret it as a way to suffuse their minds, hearts, and souls with "higher things."

The ancient tradition of meditation comes from the Latin *meditari*, meaning deep, continued reflection. Over the millennia, many types have evolved. For instance, *apophatic* meditation is designed to empty the mind by eliminating thoughts from consciousness, while the *cataphatic* focus is holding a specific image, idea, or word in the mind's eye, allowing emotions to manifest.

During the past decades, many scientific studies have verified the ways in which meditation can heal body, mind, and soul. Vipassana meditation, an ancient practice from India that was rediscovered by Gotama Buddha more than 2,500 years ago, is an especially powerful technique for food fretters. With its focus on self-transformation through self-observation, it is designed to dissolve chaotic, drifting thoughts that sabotage well-being, and instead to bring balance and peace of mind. Using the same concept of transformation through self-observation, we created a self-guided technique that we call the "food-friendly meditation." We designed it as a meditation for food fretters who are often obsessive about food and eating, and whose thoughts are filled with anxiety and judgment about food, eating, and weight. It can be a powerful tool, for meditation can change both conscious and unconscious food-related behaviors.

The Food-Friendly Meditation

Before beginning our step-by-step food-friendly meditation, look over the "What's Your Eating Style?" questionnaire, and identify the elements of food fretting with which you have the most trouble. Then, with each inhalation, imagine how each element makes you feel; with each exhalation, imagine a non–food fretting scenario. For instance:

Example: As you inhale, imagine how you feel when you are "on a diet"; exhaling, envision yourself eating tasty fresh food in a relaxed frame of mind.

Example: As you inhale, recall the guilt you feel after eating food you "shouldn't"; exhaling, delight in the flavor of a favorite food, without judgment.

Example: As you inhale, conjure up an obese person you see eating in a restaurant; exhaling, feel compassion for the person.

To obtain the full benefit, practice the following meditation fifteen to thirty minutes each day. When your mind wanders, gently bring your attention back to the imagery.

1. Set aside some time when you will not be disturbed.
2. Choose a comfortable place to sit.
3. Sit in a comfortable upright position, with relaxed shoulders.
4. Close your eyes.
5. Position your head so it is comfortably balanced between your shoulders.
6. Inhale deeply, pause for two seconds, then exhale deeply. Do this three times.
7. As you inhale, say to yourself, "I know that I am breathing in."
8. As you exhale, say to yourself, "I know that I am breathing out."

9. Identify an element of food fretting that is problematic for you, such as dieting, guilt, or judgment.

10. Inhale the problematic *situation*; exhale the *solution*.

The food-friendly meditation gives you the skills you need to let food fretting thoughts emerge, to simply observe the thoughts and behaviors, and then to let them go. The key concept: substitute the food fretting thoughts you release with opposite, positive emotions, such as acceptance, joy, pleasure, or compassion.

As you practice this meditation, keep in mind that staying focused, mindful, and in-the-moment is challenging; after all, it's easy and normal for our thoughts to wander. Because of this tendency, realize that meditation is a lifetime process. When and if you find your mind wandering, bring your thoughts back to the meditation. Your intention is to stay with the meditation as long as possible and not to perceive it as something you have to do "perfectly."

Overcoming Food Fretting

To eat—and live—optimally, consider that food is more than an amalgam of nutrients and calories that lead to weight loss—or gain. Along with healing you physically, it can improve your mood, satisfy your soul, and connect you to others and to the mystery of life. To turn food fretting–think, filled with dieting, calorie-counting, and anxious overeating, into Enlightened Diet nourishment, decide to enjoy food and the experience of eating as a social, ceremonial, sensual pleasure. This chapter gives you the insights and practical strategies you need to get started. You'll also find the slimming secrets of eating mindfully in the next chapter on the task snacking eating style to be useful tools in fighting food fretting.

Chapter 3

Task Snacking

℞: Bring moment-to-moment nonjudgmental awareness to each aspect of the meal.

Some call it "multitasking"; the French call it "vagabond eating"; in America, it's a growing trend. Whatever its form, eating a meal or snacking mindlessly while working in front of your computer, driving, watching TV, shopping with a friend, or talking on the phone, the task snacking eating style puts you at risk for overeating and becoming overweight or obese. Have you ever meandered through the mall while munching? If so, you're task snacking. Do you watch TV, flip through a magazine, or study while eating? These are more task-snacking behaviors. As a matter of fact, doing other things while you're eating has become so common in our culture, it's become normal.

Consider "car cuisine," the growing tendency for drivers to eat in their cars at drive-in restaurants or while driving. As Americans continue to eat more and more meals in their cars, food makers have accommodated the trend with what they call "cup-holder cuisine": finger-friendly foods and compact "meals" that are drop-free and glop-free. Examples include cereal bars made with dry milk; salad-in-a-cup and pancake-like breakfast sandwiches with the "yummy taste of maple syrup baked right in," available at McDonald's; squeeze tubes that contain yogurt; and drinkable soups that can be sipped from a cup. Some experts say that almost 20 percent of us consume such "meals" in cars. The trend of "dashboard dining" is so entrenched in our culture that Honda provides a pop-up table in the console, and Saab sells models with refrigerated glove boxes.[1]

However, not only do most of us not pay much attention to where we're eating, and what we're doing while we're eating, but we also don't even believe that these two factors have anything to do with our weight. But they do. We link task snacking to weight gain because our eating styles research revealed that those who were overweight task snacked more often than those who did it less often or not at all.

A Tale of Two Task Snackers

We vividly remember the moment we realized we were task snackers. We were at Heinrich-Heine, a medical university in Düsseldorf, Germany, where we had been invited to do research on lifestyle (diet, stress management, exercise, and group support) and heart disease. After several months, when we had become good friends with some colleagues, we heard a knock on our office door around lunchtime. "We're going to the cafeteria for lunch," said Siegfried. "Would you like to join us?" In response, we stopped clicking away at our computers midword, put our homemade sandwiches away, gathered our coats, and then walked through the wintry campus with three coworkers until we arrived at the building that housed the cafeteria.

In place of sitting at our desk and working at our computers while eating our sandwiches, we were greeted by students' energetic conversations as they waited in line to choose their food. After our leisurely lunch, convivial conversation, and another chance to walk and talk in the fresh, crisp air, we all returned to work. We would repeat this welcomed ritual with our friends many times during the two years we worked in Europe.

Upon reflection, I can't help but think how atypical such a social scenario has become for many Americans during lunchtime. After all, don't most of us munch mindlessly while working at our desks? One of the first studies to demonstrate the link between eating at your desk (a classic task snacking behavior) and increased risk of weight gain was done by the American Dietetic Association, which cosponsored a survey with ConAgra Foods. When they polled 1,024 full-time employees who worked at desks, they discovered that most eat while working: 67 percent eat lunch, 61 percent nibble munchies, and 37 percent eat breakfast. With an additional 10 percent of men and 7 percent of women "dining" at their desks, it seems that some continue the habit of task snacking into the evening hours.

How might desktop dining translate into an increased risk for piling on added pounds? Eating at your desk while working means you're likely to consume more food than you realize, suggests David Grotto of the American Dietetic Association.[2] Along with overeating, staying put also means you're moving less and are therefore burning fewer calories than more motion-conscious coworkers. Not surprisingly, this can lead to the tired but true formula for weight gain: eating more and moving less.

"That's exactly what happened to me," exclaimed a physician friend of ours when we told him about the link between desktop dining and weight gain. "Because I was on deadline to complete my fifth book, I ate breakfast, lunch, and dinner while working at my computer, between seeing patients," he clarified. "During this time, my wife took over my job of walking our dog each day," he added. "After nine months, I finished the manuscript; at the same time, I was surprised to discover I had gained almost twenty pounds. This had never happened to me before." Our health-savvy friend said it took almost a year to get back to his normal weight.

Anatomy of Task Snacking

Sure, it's obvious that if you're a task-snacking couch potato or mouse potato, it's likely you're not moving much. And this means that, like our friend who put on twenty pounds by being stationary for months while working on his book at his computer, lack of exercise is a key contributor to weight gain (more about this in chapter 9, "Enlightened Exercise"). But how might task snacking, specifically, work against your waistline when you eat while working, or you munch while watching TV, or you snack while driving? In other words, how may eating in a not-too-conscious, not-too-mindful way be a recipe for weight gain? Understanding what happens when you eat while task snacking provides a clue.

Because the brain can attend to only one topic at a time, when you do multiple tasks simultaneously, the mind constantly shifts its attention. If you were to undergo a PET (Positron Emission Tomography) scan—a powerful, noninvasive imaging technique that accurately images the cellular function of the human body—while task snacking, it would show lights blinking on and off in selected areas of the brain associated with the various tasks you're doing. To cope with your task snacking, when you eat while the mind is not focused on your food, the mind disengages from the body. In response, the digestive process is impaired, making food not nearly as nutritious as it could be. In turn, this malfunction can trigger hunger and malnutrition and the drive to eat more so you will feel satisfied via the nutrients both your mind and your body need for optimal health—nutrients that you're not metabolizing. In this way, task snacking can create a vicious cycle of poor digestion, inadequate nutrition, and overeating to compensate, to try to get the vitamins and minerals you're not metabolizing.

Task snacking works on yet another level: when the mind is not paying full attention to the sensation of food, such as its taste, scent, texture, and presentation (more about eating to satisfy the senses in chapter 8, "Sensory Disregard"), then eating, itself, becomes less satisfying. And a key way to compensate for getting less pleasure or gratification from food is to continue to eat . . . more and more. The bottom line? Mindless task snacking is likely to lead to eating more and enjoying it less.

In contrast, there is evidence that paying attention to food while you eat affects how your body metabolizes the food in a positive, beneficial way. Because your mind is focused solely on eating, more digestive juices, starting with your saliva, are recruited. And because eating mindfully slows down the speed with which you eat, you're also optimizing the digestive juices in your stomach; indeed, the entire digestive process is enhanced.

Can the awareness with which you eat really make a difference to your health and well-being, to the way in which you metabolize your food? Or, vice versa, does eating while task snacking actually impair your ability to absorb food?

Metabolism of Mindfulness

To find out whether eating mindfully is really beneficial to digestion, researcher Donald Morse, a physician and professor emeritus at Temple University in Philadelphia, designed a unique study to assess whether eating mindfully versus eating while distracted or stressed (task snacking) made a difference to metabolism. He designed his experiment this way: a group of female college students would meditate for five minutes before eating cereal (a food high in carbohydrates), while another group would distract themselves with mental arithmetic before eating the cereal (a form of task snacking). Afterward, when Dr. Morse and his team measured the saliva (where metabolism of food begins) of the "mindful meditators" and then compared it to that of the task snackers, he discovered, amazingly, that those who meditated mindfully before eating produced 22 percent more of the digestive enzyme alpha-amylase.

There are two interesting implications of this study. First, because alpha-amylase helps you digest and metabolize carbohydrates in carbohydrate-dense foods (such as potatoes, bread, and of course cereal), as well as B vitamins (of which there are eight), if you eat while task snacking you're likely to absorb fewer nutrients than you need for your mind-body to function optimally. It also "shows that there's a real benefit to having a leisurely meal," speculates Morse. "The decrease in alpha-amylase production is just the tip of the iceberg. When you gulp down your food, your entire digestive system is affected." And not only does task snacking have long-term implications for your digestion, but Morse's findings also imply that if you make subtle but significant changes in the awareness you bring to food and eating (meaning, when you eat, eat; when you work, work; do one thing at a time) so that you're eating mindfully, you're more likely to stop over-eating and gaining weight.[3]

Medical Meditation

If you recall, in chapter 2, "Food Fretting," I introduced you to the concept of meditation as a way to transcend this eating style. An integral aspect of world religions and Eastern healing systems (such as India's Ayurveda) for millennia, meditation initially emerged in, and penetrated, Western science in the 1970s with the publication of physician Herbert Benson's pioneering and now-classic book *The Relaxation Response*. Founding president of the Mind/Body Medical Institute at Harvard Medical School, Benson was the first person to document scientifically the deeply calming effects of meditation on the body's autonomic nervous system.

The innovative path he took to this realization is fascinating. Benson's journey began in India, where he went to do research with meditating monks in the Himalayan mountains. As part of his experiment, he placed sheets that were wet with water on the monks, who would then enter into deep meditation. The altitude was high, and the weather was freezing. Under such circumstances, most of us would expect the wet sheets to freeze, and for the monks themselves to be too uncomfortably cold to continue. But this isn't what happened. Instead, steam started to rise from the sheets that covered the meditating monks, so much so that both the sheets and the monks actually dried off without freezing or getting cold. What Benson and his team discovered from this amazing study was that with enough skill at meditation (for years, the monks' life included meditating for hours each day), human beings can control their body temperatures to an extraordinary degree. After returning to Harvard, Benson conducted more studies on the deeply calming effects of meditation. With the Harvard imprimatur, his studies led to the discovery that simple meditation techniques can profoundly calm the body's nervous system; ergo, Benson's "relaxation response" and the birth of mind-body medicine.[4]

Since Benson's findings about meditating monks in India, the field of meditation has evolved to include the practice of Medical Meditation. Proven effective by scientific studies, its unique focus is concentration, and how it can change your body, mind, and soul, and in the process bring you to a calm state of mind that holds the power to heal multi-dimensionally. And this process includes turning to mindfulness meditation to turn the tide of overeating and related weight gain. But before I tell you about groundbreaking research in the emerging field of mindfulness meditation as an antidote to task snacking and its relatives, overeating and other eating disorders, I'd like to introduce you to a more in-depth understanding of what it means to eat mindfully. As you'll see, by focusing your awareness on food and eating, you're infusing yourself with a meditative sensibility that quiets the mind, soothes the soul . . . and begins to banish binge eating.

Meet "Tea Mind"

Following Benson's work, molecular biologist Jon Kabat-Zinn created a mindfulness meditation model and program that, today, is used worldwide in institutions ranging from Kabat-Zinn's Stress Reduction Clinic at the University of Massachusetts Medical Center to hundreds of hospitals and clinics, corporations, sports teams, and prisons. A meditator himself since 1966, Kabat-Zinn created his technique to give people an experiential, hands-on sense of what it means to meditate mindfully. And patients, who have been referred to his clinic for ailments ranging from stress to heart disease, reap the rewards with a unique Buddhist-based meditation structured by Kabat-Zinn around the ordinary experience of eating; he calls it the "raisin meditation."

As Kabat-Zinn guides participants through his raisin meditation, they focus on all aspects of the experience of eating one simple raisin: how it looks, smells, and feels; what happens in the mouth before, during, and after eating it; the motion and movement involved; the raisin's taste and texture; swallowing; and the role of breathing throughout the experience. From start to finish, it takes ten minutes to eat the sole raisin. And then the group is ready to begin the mindfulness raisin meditation process again with the second raisin everyone is holding.[5]

Later in this chapter, I'll guide you through this meditation (see "Raisin Consciousness"), but for now the key concept for you to get is the "consciousness" behind it: eating with moment-to-moment, nonjudgmental attention to each element of the entire experience. What does it mean to have such focused attention on food? Is it simply paying attention to the ordinary experience of eating? Or is it something more extraordinary? Or is it mundane? Ancient food wisdom that has served humankind for millennia offers some clues about what it means to be aware of being aware.

I vividly remember the moment I was introduced to the Chinese idea of "tea mind." It was during a visit to the Urasenke Foundation in San Francisco, where I had been invited to observe students studying the Japanese Way of Tea (*chanoyu*). At any one time, I heard the pouring of water, the clink of the lid on the iron kettle, or the whisking of the powdered green tea in water as it turned into a light, frothy brew. Surrounded by *chanoyu*'s timeless refinement, I realized that as much as it is an actual ceremony, it is also a consciousness, a "mentality of elegance," an experiential adventure that unfolds along with the passing moments. Creating the alchemical brew with such a consciousness is also a path to tea mind. With roots in Taoism, it means that, like tea, a person's mind is limitless and a part of everything. And, as with the raisin meditation, accessing tea mind calls for drinking tea using all your senses, and more.[6]

While Taoism provided the aesthetic ideals inherent in the Way of Tea, it was a southern Zen Buddhist sect that integrated many Taoist doctrines into Japan's Way of Tea as it is practiced today. Nowhere is this appreciation of aesthetics more evident than in the placement of flowers, the profound simplicity of the pottery, the architecture of the teahouse, and of course the tea powder itself. So integral is a refined consciousness to the Way of Tea in Japanese culture that the concept has infiltrated the language through the word *chajin*, which describes a person who has internalized the meditative awareness inherent in tea mind. Observe the visible and invisible elements as they play together to satisfy the senses, and notice the tea mind infusion that makes you less prone to overeat, in place of the busyness inherent in task snacking.

A Feel-Good Feedback Loop

Can the ephemeral, meditative sensibility inherent in the "unseeable principles" of tea mind and meditation make a difference to your weight and well-being? And if so, in what way? To answer these questions, researchers have begun to delve into the ancient discipline of mindfulness meditation to explore its potential to manage eating disorders. The idea to turn to meditation therapy as a treatment option for eating disorders has its roots in the growing field of brain research. In one of the first scientific studies done in the late 1960s on the meditating brain, psychiatrist Gregg Jacobs, of Harvard Medical School, recorded the EEGs (brain waves) of meditators and another group of subjects who had been given books on tape to listen to as a way to relax. Over the next few months, Jacobs noted that the meditators had lower activity in the parietal lobe section of the brain; when this sensory section of the brain shuts down, it's possible to feel fewer "boundaries" and in turn to feel more connected to, and one with, the universe.[7]

The underlying mechanism: the meditating brain doesn't literally shut down; rather, it slows the receipt of information and keeps it from entering the parietal lobe, the part of the brain that orients us to time and space. Still more brain-imaging studies by Richard Davidson at the University of Wisconsin at Madison revealed that when you meditate regularly, the brain reorients from a right, prefrontal-oriented mindset of stress and discontent to a left-prefrontal disposition of relaxation and joy.[8] This reorientation is intriguing in terms of task snacking because it explains how your brain produces the relaxation response Benson discovered when you meditate; it is also yet another perspective about the profound way in which eating mindfully reduces stress and, in turn, lowers the odds of overeating.

Meditation for Managing Binge Eating

What does mindfulness and meditation have to do with eating, task snacking, and your weight? A lot. In our research on the seven eating styles, the more that study participants reduced their task snacking, the more they reduced their weight, suggesting that you eat less when you focus more on your food and the process of eating than when you eat while task snacking. The field of psychology is in its infancy in doing experiments that demonstrate the impact of mindfulness meditation and its link to less overeating and more weight loss, but there are some examples. Let me give you three of them.

There is a wonderful study of putting mindfulness meditation into action as a way to reduce overeating and obesity. In the 1980s Jean Kristeller of Indiana State University, where she is a professor of psychology and director of the Center for the Study of Health, Religion, and Spirituality, began to use meditation first to help patients de-stress with Benson's relaxation response; then, inspired by Kabat-Zinn's raisin meditation, she turned her attention to meditation as a vehicle to help people with compulsive eating problems. Over time, she developed her Mindfulness-Based Eating Awareness Training (MB-EAT), a comprehensive nine-week program that integrates the experience of food and eating with "inner" and "outer" wisdom. It is replete with meditative exercises that address hunger and satiety, forgiveness, and connecting to the inner wisdom that signals whether you're full and satisfied or hungry with an appetite for a particular food. MB-EAT's key focus is finding satisfaction in quality, not quantity.

To find out whether her MB-EAT program could help women with eating and weight problems, Kristeller recruited eighteen obese women, aged twenty-five to sixty-two, each of whom met the American Psychiatric Association's *Diagnostic and Statistical Manual of Mental Disorders* (DSM-IV) criteria for Binge Eating Disorder (BED), which is defined as recurrent episodes of out-of-control eating twice a week or more for six months or longer. The actual intervention focused on three forms of meditation: general mindfulness meditation, eating meditation, and mini-meditations. With the general meditation, participants were taught to develop focused attention and awareness of an object, such as food. They would do this simply by noting thoughts, emotions, or bodily sensations as they arose, then returning their attention to their breath when they noticed their thoughts were straying. This particular practice teaches individuals to observe the contents of the mind and the sensations of the body, without judgment, and at the same time to learn detached awareness. The eating meditation applies the general mindfulness meditation approach to more specific behaviors, beliefs, and emotions associated with food intake; again, emphasis is on retaining detached awareness. To do meditations, participants were instructed to take a few moments to stop and become aware of their thoughts and feelings prior to meals, or when the urge to binge surfaces.

After learning these techniques, participants met once a week for a period of six weeks. For the first twenty minutes of each session, they discussed progress and any difficulties they may have experienced during the prior week. Next, they focused on a specific theme related to overcoming binge eating, such as becoming aware of binge triggers, hunger and satiety, self-forgiveness, and relapse prevention, using exercises in eating mindfully. Homework between sessions included daily meditation, either on tape or self-guided, and mindful-eating exercises.

At the end of the six weeks, Kristeller concluded that the six-week program was, indeed, beneficial. Three weeks prior to starting the intervention, most women binged an average of five times each week. But after three weeks of learning and practicing mindfulness meditation in preparation for the study, the women lowered their average number of bingeing episodes to 3.9. And when the six week program ended, the average number of binges was less than one (.9) per week.[9] Just as encouraging, when Kristeller did a three-week follow-up, she discovered the women were still benefiting, with bingeing episodes less than twice (1.6) weekly. In other words, bingeing behavior continued after the study, but the number of episodes was much fewer than when the study started. Significantly, emotions that often sparked a bingeing episode, such as depression and anxiety, decreased. Kristeller's findings were so encouraging that the Center for Complementary and Alternative Medicine at the National Institutes of Health funded the psychologist and her team at Duke University to do a similar nine-week program. The focus of her next study is to examine how mindfulness meditation can promote weight loss.[10]

Upon reflection, it may seem paradoxical that as the women in Kristeller's study let go of trying to control their eating, it led to more control over their binge eating in terms of doing it less often. A possible explanation is that when you do mindfulness meditation, you learn to detach yourself from the random impulse to binge and then to act on it by eating. In other words, mindfulness meditation empowers you to disconnect that circuit in the brain that attaches an emotion with a certain behavior sequence (bingeing). This suggests that if you have a negative feeling and want to binge, when you do mindfulness meditation, you put space between your feelings and bingeing; you realize that feelings come and go and you don't necessarily have to act on them. In this way, you obtain a sense of control over bingeing and are empowered to turn to it as a coping mechanism less often. But the question still remains: If you focus your attention through meditation, can it lead to weight loss? Will research that explores this question expose meditation as an effective antidote to the task snacking and related weight gain with which so many of us struggle?

Meditation and Your Weight

A first-of-its kind study that sheds light on the meditation/weight equation was conducted by researchers at Dr. Dean Ornish's Preventive Medicine Research Institute (PMRI) in Sausalito, California. The study, which has its roots in work Ornish did throughout the 1980s and 1990s, put meditation on the map when he included it as part of a comprehensive lifestyle program that showed you can reverse heart disease through lifestyle changes alone—stress management (meditation and yoga); a no-fat-added plant-based diet; exercise; and group support—without drugs or surgery. Ornish's research was pioneering because it was substantive and sound and published in prestigious medical journals, ranging from the *Journal of the American Medical Association* to *The Lancet* and other peer-reviewed journals.[11]

Since the publication of Ornish's reversal research, many health professionals have contacted him over the years wanting to know which components of the program contributed the most to reversing heart disease. Was it the low-fat diet? Or the stress management techniques? Perhaps it was the exercise? Or could it be the group support? Or was it the combination of all the components, working synergistically, that brought the benefits? Ornish and his research team decided to find out. "Clearly, a study testing each component separately would offer much-needed information that could help many," medical psychologist Gerdi Weidner, PhD, told me. I talked with Weidner, vice president and director of research at PMRI, to learn about the results of the study firsthand. Formerly a professor of psychology and preventive medicine at the State University of New York at Stony Brook, Weidner met the coauthor of this book, Larry Scherwitz, in 1992 in Hannover, Germany, where he was presenting the Ornish reversal program at the International Society of Behavioral Medicine Conference. Scherwitz was presenting the lifestyle research because he had been Ornish's director of research for more than fifteen years—prior to Weidner taking over the position. At the time of his presentation, Scherwitz and I were living in Germany, replicating Ornish's lifestyle research at a 350-bed clinic; my role was director of nutrition.

Continued Weidner: "With more than 850 patients with heart disease (both male and female) who have been enrolled in the Ornish program for at least three months, we now have a great opportunity to investigate the individual and joint contribution of lifestyle changes to coronary risk factors that are recommended by the Ornish program. In our new study, the Multi-Site Cardiac Lifestyle Intervention Program (MCLIP), we studied these patients in order to investigate the degree to which changing one's lifestyle behaviors (lowering dietary fat and increasing exercise and stress management practices of meditation and yoga) can improve risk factors linked with heart disease, such as weight, cholesterol levels, and depression and hostility." To do this, patients and their spouses met in groups for three months, Weider told me, during which time they got together twice weekly, for a total of 104 hours, to learn about the low-fat diet, exercise, and stress management techniques, which included yoga sessions that ended with about ten minutes of meditation. During their non-meeting time, participants were asked to practice stress management for one hour per day, and they were given the option of doing this by listening to meditation tapes.[12]

Not surprisingly, results revealed all three intervention modalities (diet, stress management, and exercise) played a positive role in lowering risk factors for heart disease. For task snackers, though, what is most relevant about the study are three key findings: The first reveals that *the amount of time each person spent meditating was directly linked with the amount of weight that was lost, regardless of whether participants changed their dietary fat intake or their exercise habits.* Indeed, those who did *not* change their dietary fat intake, but increased their stress management practice by as much as six hours per week, lost an average of almost twenty pounds (men) and more than twelve pounds (women). Second, as pertinent, the greatest weight loss was achieved by those who *increased* their yoga and meditation, while they *decreased* their intake of dietary fat. Specifically, those who increased their stress management practice to six hours per week *and* reduced their dietary fat intake to 15 percent calories-from-fat lost an average of about twenty-seven pounds (men) and twenty pounds (women) at the end of three months. The third key finding goes against conventional energy-in (food), energy-out (exercise) guidelines we discussed in chapter 2, "Food Fretting": in the Multi-Site Cardiac Lifestyle Intervention Program, an increase in exercise did *not* contribute any further to the amount of weight loss. Rather, it was the amount of time participants meditated, and the degree to which they lowered their dietary fat intake, that brought the best results.

Although the exact reasons stress management leads to weight loss are unclear, Weidner offers several possible explanations about why meditation may contribute to weight loss. First, meditation directs your awareness away from external cues (such as eating lunch at noon, when you "should") to focusing your attention internally (eating when you're actually feeling hungry). Second, it may also diminish stress-related eating (the next chapter on "Emotional Eating" discusses this in detail), turning to food when you're feeling anxious or upset.

What is especially relevant to the Enlightened Diet and the seven eating styles is what Ornish always says: practicing all components of his program is the key to achieving beneficial health outcomes—including weight loss. And he is right. Adds Weidner: "In our analyses, increases in stress management and meditation contributed not only to weight loss but also to reductions in diabetic risk and hostile feelings [a risk factor for heart disease]. And less dietary fat intake added further to weight loss and to reductions in perceived stress. Add exercise to the equation, and your ability to burn energy (calories) increases."[13] So, too, with the Enlightened Diet: optimize and implement all of the antidotes to the eating styles discussed in *The Enlightened Diet*, including eating mindfully, and you're more likely to lose more weight.

Raisin Consciousness

From yoga to Hinduism to Buddhism, hundreds of types of meditation from the East have evolved over the millennia. Over the past few decades, more and more of these techniques have been integrated into mind-body medicine, a growing field of Western medical care. The practice and cultivation of mindful awareness is rooted in one of Buddhism's earliest sutras, ancient Buddhist teachings. Called the Mindfulness Sutra, it describes how to cultivate judgment-free, impartial awareness of what you are doing during each moment. The raisin meditation that Jon Kabat-Zinn imparts to his patients is based on ancient Buddhist wisdom he learned from Jack Kornfield, one of the key Buddhist teachers in the West. Here is a version that you can experience for yourself. To get the most benefit from it, first read through it, then do it.

1. Sit in a comfortable chair and set a small bowl filled with raisins next to you on a table.
2. Select one raisin from the bowl.
3. Look at the raisin as if it were an alien object you had never seen before.
4. As you look at the raisin, imagine it in its original form as a grape, growing in the sunshine surrounded by air, earth, and water.
5. Continuing to look at the raisin, describe what you see: its texture, color, and shape, and anything else that comes to mind.
6. Bring the raisin up to your nose. Smell it. Describe its scent.
7. As you smell the raisin, are you experiencing any changes in your mouth, in your saliva, as you anticipate eating the raisin?

continued

8. How does the raisin feel? Describe it.

9. Become aware of your body and the hand that is holding the raisin. Consider how your hand knows how to hold the raisin, how to bring it up toward your nose.

10. Bring the raisin toward your lips, then place it in your mouth. What motion is your tongue doing? Your jaw? Your teeth? Your cheek?

11. Now, put all your attention into your mouth. As you do, bite into the raisin . . . slowly . . . and begin to chew . . . slowly. Stop chewing after three chews. On which side of your mouth are you chewing? What motion are your tongue, jaw, teeth, and cheek doing now?

12. Describe the taste you're experiencing.

13. Now, continue to chew, but do not swallow the raisin. Do you notice a difference in the taste? What is the texture like?

14. Are you tempted to swallow yet? Observe what is happening in your mouth as you prepare to swallow. Now, swallow the raisin. Then imagine it in your stomach, and acknowledge that your body is one raisin heavier.

15. Can you "taste" your breath now? Focus your attention on your breath, as you inhale and exhale . . . slowly.

16. Remain focused on your breath as you continue to inhale and exhale. Now, simply become silent.

If your mind wanders, once you notice this is happening, bring your attention back to your breath. For the next five, ten, or fifteen minutes, or longer, continue to focus on your breathing.

Congratulations! You have just experienced mindfulness meditation. To reap the rewards, meditating twenty to thirty minutes each day is optimal. If setting aside some special time to meditate is challenging for you, consider turning each meal or snack into an opportunity to eat mindfully. Later in this book (chapter 10, "In Action"), I'll guide you through a step-by-step seven-eating-styles meditation that will give you the skills you need to put the Enlightened Diet into action each time you eat. But for now, take a cue from time-tested ancient food wisdom: pay attention to every food-related act, every sensation and perception, for its own sake, to stay in the moment. From planning and preparing a meal, to serving, eating, and cleanup, regardless of which stage or stages of the meal on which you choose to focus, take your actions off autopilot and, instead, commit to being fully aware of what your hands, mouth, and mind are experiencing moment to moment. For in the witnessing lies the antidote to task snacking.

Other Simple Strategies

Cultivating mindfulness—paying attention intentionally—empowers you to slow down long enough to experience the subtleties of food. This awareness is beneficial because when you focus on your food, you're not task snacking; you're simply tasting your food and savoring the experience of eating. In chapter 8, "Sensory Disregard," I'll tell you more about the power of the time-tested nutrition philosophy of the "six tastes" espoused by Eastern healing systems, such as India's Ayurveda medicine, traditional Chinese medicine (TCM), and Tibetan Medicine. Right now, though, you can reap the rewards by focusing on the flavors in food each time you eat.

Savor flavor. The next time you eat a mixed meal, such as a salad or stew made with varied ingredients, bring your attention to your mouth; then, as you chew your food, try to identify the flavors in your food. For instance, is it mostly sweet, or is salt the major flavor? Did you experience a burst of flavor at the first bite? Are you still enjoying the taste of the food after the second and third bites?

Take tea time. Another way to approach your journey of mindfulness is to perceive tea as an opportunity to balance the five elements of metal (minerals in the soil that help create tea leaves); wood (the tea plant); water (that brews and brings tea back to life); fire (the sun that heats the water); and earth (the mother of tea and material for tea pots). Followers of Japan's Way of Tea (often called the Japanese Tea Ceremony) believe that when the elements are balanced and in harmony, they create a form of perfection. The next time you take time to savor some tea, can you see and taste each element with each sip? Consider bringing a similar tea consciousness to all beverages you consume during the day, such as water, juice, coffee, or milk.

Move into mindfulness. There are three distinct steps to take to move into mindfulness and replace task snacking with conscious, intentional awareness: (1) Intentionality: don't just think about doing it; make a decisive choice to focus on the food before you when you're eating; (2) Commitment: act on your intention, and carry it out, by gently letting go of feelings, thoughts, and activities that may be interfering with your intention and commitment to mindfulness; and (3) Focus: with intention and commitment to mindfulness, keep your attention on the food or food-related activities.

Overcoming Task Snacking

Taking the time to enjoy food, to truly taste and savor it, is the key to overcoming task snacking and reducing the odds of weight gain. Replace eating while doing other things, such as walking, working, or watching television, with moment-to-moment nonjudgmental awareness of each aspect of your meal, and you're on the path of the Enlightened Diet. The next chapter, on emotional eating, reveals another facet of the Enlightened Diet. As you'll see, it builds on techniques of mindfulness, while giving you more insights into the skills you need to win at weight loss.

Chapter 4

Emotional Eating

℞ : Eat only for pleasure and when you're feeling feel-good feelings.

In the twenty-five-plus years that Barbara Birsinger has been studying emotional eating, she has come to believe that emotional eaters seek food in an attempt to manage unpleasant feelings, such as depression, anxiety, or anger. In other words, when negative emotions emerge, emotional eaters turn to food as a distraction, as a way to run away from, and to numb, these feelings. They are not eating because they are hungry; they are eating in response to disagreeable emotions and feelings.

Birsinger knows a lot about emotional eating—both personally and as a professional who is a registered dietitian (RD) with a doctorate in theology, spiritual healing, and energy medicine. Her epiphany came from her own early struggles with emotional eating, which developed into an eating disorder that she successfully overcame. Her insights emerged a few years after she graduated from the University of California, Berkeley, where she obtained a master's degree in public health nutrition. Emotional eating—and overcoming it—means so much to her that it was the focus of the research she did for her dissertation.

How did Birsinger win her battle with emotional eating? When I talked with her, she told me that she didn't want to live her life focused on food and feelings. She wanted a balanced life that included marriage and children, both of which have been a part of her life for many years. I am convinced that her profound compassion for the millions who struggle with food and weight, and her deep interest in nutrition and optimal eating, had a lot to do with her personal success.

During our discussion, Birsinger told me about her personal experience with her own food- and weight-related struggles; she also revealed a lot about her research on overcoming emotional eating and overeating. I wanted to speak with Birsinger, specifically, because we share a strong conviction that optimal eating and normal weight aren't achieved via a list of "do and don't" instructions; they are the side effects that come naturally when you perceive food and eating as a path that leads to physical, emotional, spiritual, and social well-being; in other words, your relationship with food and eating is transformed from a problem into a solution when you allow food to heal you in every way.

Our total talk time took a little over six hours. The excerpt of our conversation that follows is just a fraction of the story Birsinger shared with concern and care. Her insights are especially useful because I think they provide a clear portrait of how she transformed a life of emotional eating and yo-yo weight problems into one that is based on a solid foundation of mind-body balance.

> There was a lot of love in my family and thankfully I always knew that. But along with an abundance of love, there was an abundance of food. I grew up on a farm in the Midwest. My father was a veterinarian, and my mother, a housewife in the 1950s, gardened, cooked, baked, and canned. Food was plentiful and always available, and there were few rules around it. We ate three meals a day of delicious, fresh, homemade food, which included our own homegrown meats and dairy, and fresh fruits and vegetables. We could snack freely on freshly baked bread, fruit pies, and cookies, all of which were stocked in a huge pantry to which I had easy access.

My father died of a long illness when I was a child, and his death was a taboo topic. Growing up in a family that didn't acknowledge feelings, I experienced considerable emotional stress. We moved from the farm at the time I started middle school, and this is when I started to develop a problem with food and body image. In junior high school, I was teased about being too skinny; after all, people were judging how I looked all the time. My girlfriend and I decided to eat double lunches to gain weight, but we just got taller, not more curvy.

We moved again, this time to an affluent community, just when I started high school, and it was lonely. I didn't know anybody and felt that I didn't fit in. I gained twenty-five pounds in the first year. About this time, I met a girl who was dieting, so I decided to try it, too. I rode my bike seven miles to school each day, surviving on lettuce, and yes, I lost weight. It amazed me that no one noticed or was aware of the danger I was putting myself in with constant dieting and fasting. At the same time, I studied hard and I liked school, but I hated the social and competitive aspects of high school, so I graduated in three years, instead of four. This meant that I started UC, Berkeley, at sixteen, and being younger than the other students and emotionally unprepared, college was stressful, and I wasn't prepared emotionally; and as with high school, it was lonely and isolating.

By the time I was eighteen, I had been dieting for several years. Now I started to get gastric reflux symptoms: food wouldn't digest and it would start to come up through my esophagus. After many doctor visits, and not being able to stop the reflux, I began to use it as a weight control method, and later I started to binge eat. My bingeing was related to the emotional issues I was going through. It was hard for me to stomach the stress of being so young at a huge university, and having inadequate emotional support at school and at home, I was stuffing down my feelings; after all, I was taught to keep them in with the hope that they would go away; there just weren't any other acceptable choices in my family.

When I started thinking about how to stop binge eating, I realized that when I felt upset or anxious, food helped to calm me down and to feel better. When I felt overwhelmed by my emotions, it felt like a tidal wave, and I would binge to cope. The foods I binged on were foods that had been abundant in our home while I was growing up: scrumptious cinnamon twists, homemade bread with butter and jam, chocolate chip cookies, and apple and peach pies.

Then, when I was about twenty-six, I sat down in silence one day out of deep despair with my situation. I knew I wanted to stop. I wanted a different life. I didn't want to feel like an imposter with a secret life anymore. It was in the seventies, and I had gone to therapists, but at the time, they didn't know about emotional eating or eating disorders yet, and the doctors I saw couldn't help either. I realized that inevitably, it was up to me and me alone to help myself.

When I looked at the pattern of everything that contributed to my bingeing, clearly the emotional component was the strongest reason. Binges were in response to emotions and feelings I wasn't capable of dealing with in the moment, and bingeing was how I would get relief. I had spent ten years running from feelings I realized I could actually live through without bingeing. Another turning point was identifying the amount of food I could eat without having a reflux response. Then I decided to start eating without bingeing, which included stocking shelves with all of the foods that I grew up with—many of which had become illegal by dieting standards or unhealthy according to nutrition textbooks. It was liberating to know that I didn't have to eat all the food at once because I could trust my body with the amount it wanted, and I could have it again, anytime. Knowing this, I might have some more of whatever it was I wanted within an hour or two after eating, but most often I didn't want more.

In retrospect, I realize I was relearning what we now call Intuitive Eating. I was learning to tune in to internal cues to guide me to know whether I was eating because I was hungry, or if I had an appetite for a particular food, or if I was satiated and no longer really wanted to eat. We're all born with the ability to eat this way, to look within to know what our mind and body need and want, and how much to eat; to be with yourself and your feelings and not stuff them down with food. I also stopped exercising compulsively to keep my weight down if I overate. I wanted to be healthy and to have an active life with children and grandchildren. Not to get rid of calories. I wanted to end the eating disorders way more than I was concerned about being fat. It was then that I began working on emotional and spiritual issues.[1]

Why was Birsinger able to take a sudden intuitive leap of understanding and transform a ten-year habit of emotional eating into normal, optimal eating? How, exactly, did she create such profound, meaningful change in her relationship to food, eating, and weight— changes that stayed with her for life? And if Birsinger can do it, can the millions of us who struggle with the same issues have the same success? Birsinger's transformation gives us clues about how to change, while her research on the topic, discussed later in the chapter, provides empirical evidence that decoding your emotions is the key to success. But first, let's visit the world of emotional eaters, those who have successfully left it, and the science that supported their journey.

Feeding Negative Feelings with Food

For Ann, nighttime binge eating starts after work with a trip to the supermarket to buy bags of corn chips and chunks of her favorite chocolate. Then she heads home, changes into comfortable clothes, and turns on the TV. Settling into bed surrounded by her favorite foods, she begins what she describes as "zoning out"—eating until she feels calmer— often to the point of falling in and out of sleep well before bedtime.

Although this is a typical evening for Ann, three hours after starting her binge, she is amazed to find that she has finished all the food. On a not-quite-conscious level, she senses the chips and chocolate allay her anxiety in some way. She's also concerned about these binges because she wants to lose fifty pounds and stop zoning out, but she hasn't figured out how to accomplish this. Dieting hasn't helped, nor has willpower or the techniques she's read about in self-help books. In the meantime, Ann remains vaguely depressed and distressed, and dependent on food binges to manage her darker moods.

From hard-core drugs to food, theories have abounded for decades about the causes of all kinds of chemical and behavioral addictions. Cassandra Vieten, PhD, is a clinical psychologist and researcher who specializes in mind-body medicine and behavioral disorders at California Pacific Medical Center Research Institute in San Francisco and at the Institute of Noetic Sciences in nearby Petaluma. She believes "negative affect" may be the unifying factor in overeating, disordered eating, or a growing dependency on an addiction to food influenced by genetics, environment, brain chemistry, and family dynamics. "Negative affect is distress that can be conscious or unconscious, physiological, emotional, psychological, and/or spiritual," Vieten told me. "Distress is part of life, but some experience greater amounts of it, or are more highly sensitive to it due to their hardwiring or upbringing. Others experience stress as intolerable because they haven't developed the capacity to endure negative feelings." Indeed, our research on the Enlightened Diet, which revealed the seven eating styles that form it, showed that negative emotions—especially depression, boredom, and frustration—are the feelings that drive impulse eating and cravings; indeed, they are the strongest predictor of overeating and ensuing overweight and obesity.

Bad, worrisome, anxious, unpleasant feelings are clearly a key aspect of negative affect for many, but for others—such as Ann, who fixates on food for less conscious reasons—suppressed, unexpressed, or unidentified feelings can also be part of the negative affect picture that may manifest in emotional eating. "Some people can't or won't express themselves even when they know they are experiencing fear or anger. Still others often feel nondescript distress, but they can't say why, nor can they put a name on it," said Vieten.

When a person experiences undifferentiated negative affect, it may convey itself through bodily sensations, such as a tight stomach or muscular tension. If ongoing or extreme, these physical feelings can translate into a sense that you're not going to survive the emotions. Unfortunately, many treat (self-medicate) these sensations by overeating certain foods that actually alter their mental state. Because overeating can halt the distress—for the moment—it can become a powerful reinforcer. But there's a caveat: it's possible to build up a tolerance, and to need more and more food to feel good again. When this happens, you're not really eating to feel better; you may be bingeing just to feel normal. The good news is there are also ways to build your tolerance to distress—ways to relate to it, contain it, and cope with it, so that you are less and less driven to engage in self-medicating behaviors.[2]

Of Food and Mood

Although the term "emotional eating" wasn't in the culture in 1960 when Overeaters Anonymous (OA) was founded, "HALT" was already in use by Alcoholics Anonymous and was borrowed by OA. An organization that offers a twelve-step recovery program for compulsive overeating and other eating disorders, OA warned its members early on against becoming too Hungry, too Angry, too Lonely, or too Tired because when you're feeling HALT emotions and you're an overeater, such emotions may trigger a binge. Feeling HALT emotions means you are more likely to seek *false* relief by abusing yourself with food: become too hungry, and too many cookies may override healthful food choices; chomping on chips may suppress anger; ice cream may soothe loneliness; or you may befriend french fries when you feel tired. Whatever the emotional upset, in place of giving (gifting?)

yourself what you really need, you choose food and compulsive over-eating as your solution.

OA was way ahead of its time—and science—when it linked HALT emotions with the tendency for overeaters to turn to food for comfort. Today, health professionals often use the term "self-medicate" to describe the drive behind eating to cope and to feel better when unpleasant emotions such as depression and anxiety emerge.

The idea that the food you eat can actually medicate your mood and vice versa—that your mood may motivate you to make certain food choices—was given the scientific stamp of approval in the 1970s when Judith Wurtman, PhD, a scientist at the Massachusetts Institute of Technology, revealed a fascinating facet of the emotional eating enigma. Call it nutritional neuroscience, psychoneuroimmunology, the study of food and mood, or psychological nutrition (our term for it), Wurtman launched a new field of pioneering nutrition research that has confirmed what OA and many of us know intuitively: what you eat affects your mind and mood, your tendency to pile on pounds, even the quality of your life.

When Wurtman and her husband, Richard Wurtman, MD, also at MIT, first linked food with mood, it was based on their discovery that naturally occurring sugar and starch in carbohydrate foods (such as potatoes and whole grains), as well as sugar that is added to food products (such as cookies and cake), elevate a powerful, naturally occurring chemical in your brain called serotonin. Even more fascinating was their discovery about the impact serotonin and other neurotransmitters (substances that pass information from cell to cell in the brain) have on your every mood, emotion, and food craving. For instance, about twenty minutes after you eat a carbohydrate-rich food, your brain releases serotonin; in turn, you feel more relaxed and calm. Want to feel more perky? Consume a lean, high-protein food, such as fish, and the substance that's released (norepinephrin) will let you feel more awake and energetic (unlike the kick you get from caffeine, though, you're not stimulated, just more alert).[3]

Now here is where the food-mood link really gets interesting. Since the Wurtmans' research, we've had strong clinical evidence that carbohydrates can be calming; protein-based foods can perk you up; and certain fats in food end up as endorphins, substances in the brain that produce pleasurable feelings. But now we also know that the sugary and sweet, or crunchy and fried, *processed food products* emotional eaters most often choose to get a serotonin high and to feel more relaxed, contribute to *deficiencies* in certain vitamins and minerals (nutrients) that can cause your emotions to plummet, causing you to have a serious case of depression doldrums. In this way, the food-mood syndrome becomes a vicious emotional cycle: You're feeling down, so you binge on, say, a prepackaged brownie. Sure, the brownie's sugar and white flour carb content will soothe you and calm you down, but the high sugar content of the brownie has a hidden side effect: it actually depletes some nutrients in your body that, when you have enough, could combat depression. The sweet concoction may somehow soothe your soul, but isn't it ironic that at the same time, it may also contribute to your anxiety, depression, and other unpleasant emotions? To bust the blues with food, look over the "'B' Wise" tips toward the end of this chapter.

Tapping into Transformation

While most of us try to cope with our emotions, food, and weight with the food fretting eating style—dieting, counting calories or carbs, measuring portion size, restricting or avoiding foods, and continuing to worry about our weight—those who transition successfully, permanently, and effectively from emotional eating to optimal eating and weight, as Barbara Birsinger did, reject food fretting. Instead, they tap into their emotions, they identify their real needs, and then they act on what would satisfy those needs. Often, what brings true satisfaction has nothing to do with food, although sometimes it does.

There is an excellent example of the life-transforming dynamics that allowed Birsinger to stop food fretting and bingeing, and transition from being an emotional eater to an optimal eater, in the work of Eckhart Tolle, author of *The Power of Now*. Prior to his complete change, he lived as a hermit, immersed in a depressed and anxiety-filled frame of mind; his emotional pain was so all-invasive that he considered ending his life. And then, at the depth of his despair, he realized that his miserable self, and the "I," the "owner" of his miserable self, weren't two different people; that only the "I" was real. Fully conscious and stunned at this realization, he felt "intense fear," so much so that he began to shake. At the same time, he was guided to "resist nothing," and instead to become one with simply being alive. And then he fell into a deep sleep. The next morning, Tolle awakened filled with a deep understanding and appreciation of life itself, and the wonder of his existence. Something profoundly transcendent had happened to him.

Tolle was so immersed in his bliss he spent two years living on park benches, simply *being* "in a state of the most intense joy." It was during this time he realized that regardless of ever-changing circumstances, situations, or emotions—whether positive or negative, happy or sad, good or bad, painful or joyful—he lives with an underlying sense of peace, calmness, and connection to a larger whole; that the "mystery of life," if you will, is constant. And this realization is what gave him—and continues to give him—deep peace of mind.[4]

It sounds so simple, doesn't it? Just access the truth that is within you to transform emotions that lead to overeating into a blissful, peaceful life without weight worries. As you know and I know, for most of us, making a lightening quick shift in your way of being and seeing the world is neither instant, nor is it easy. Rather, changing from being *in* the world and feeding your emotions with food, to being *of* the world and *feeling* your connection to food and eating or any other joy-filled, intentionally chosen activity, is often a messy process that starts with small steps and lots of contemplation before you can take action.

What made Barbara Birsinger able to transform and grow herself from being an emotional eater into a normal eater? Obviously, whether suddenly, or slowly and over time, she was able to let go of and move beyond a limited sense of self and expand the vision of her purpose, destiny, and role in the universe. What especially sets her apart is that instead of accepting her eating disorder as is, she was transformed when she felt passionate about moving beyond what she was *doing*, and instead, somehow, she knew she needed to *be* part of something bigger than herself. For Birsinger, this larger connection meant healing so she could become a wife and mother, and to do this called for learning to *be* outside herself and be other-oriented. In other words, by integrating and connecting her emotions, thoughts, dreams, and visions with the outside world, a spark was ignited that enabled her to launch a transformation that led to a more fulfilling, balanced, meaningful life.

Vieten offers this insight into transformation as a means to end emotional eating: "Connecting to something deeper than your individual craving or desire can also be incredibly helpful. Not only can it empower you to ride the waves of craving, emotional and spiritual awareness can enable you to use intention and choice to decide how you want to live in the world."[5]

Evolution of Emotional Eating

The specialty of emotional eating has come a long way since the 1960s when Overeaters Anonymous advised its members to HALT negative feelings of Hunger, Anger, Loneliness, and Tiredness.[6] Since then, a comprehensive emotional eating industry has evolved, replete with sound research, support groups, therapy options, and books. Barbara Birsinger didn't have these choices when she was a teenager and college student in the 1970s, struggling alone with emotional eating and other eating disorders. She recalls that during this time some early clues began to emerge about emotional eating and other eating disorders, clues that eating disorders were coming out of the closet and into the culture.

Chocolate: Elixir of Love

No discussion about emotional eating, food and mood, and weight would be complete without pausing to savor the emotional ambrosia that is associated with choice chocolate. For centuries, it has been lauded in literature, has been christened "food of the gods" with its botanical name (*theobroma-cacao*), and has flourished as an aphrodisiac. Today, the art of chocolate continues to manifest in movies such as *Charlie and the Chocolate Factory*, Laura Esquival's *Like Water for Chocolate*, the 2001 Academy Award nominee *Chocolat*, and the famous line from *Forrest Gump*, "Life is like a box of chocolates, you never know what you're gonna get." But as science continues to focus its microscope on chocolate, the more and more we *do* know what we're gonna get: emotional gratification and physical nourishment.

Today, science is verifying that chocolate offers more than alleged aphrodisiac powers and that it does, indeed, nourish both mind and body. The sugar, fat, and caffeine content of today's chocolate confections, combined with some of cocoa's naturally occurring chemicals, holds the power both to enhance your emotions and, perhaps, even heal the heart. Consider what happens when you consume the sweet-and-creamy concoction of cocoa combined with sugar and fat: blues-busting *endorphins*, naturally occurring substances (hormones) in the brain that function as painkillers and produce pleasurable feelings, are released. Such mood enhancers are compounded by the *phenylethylamine* (PEA) in chocolate, a substance that likely enhances the release of endorphins. Indeed, the PEA that is released when you eat chocolate is the same PEA that produces its euphoric side effects when you fall in love. Add druglike constituents in chocolate like caffeine and phenylethylamine, and you may have a recipe for "chocoholism."

Just as interesting is recent research about good quality *dark* chocolate (which contains a high percentage of cocoa) recently presented at the European Society of Cardiology in Munich. Apparently, dark chocolate's high levels of flavonoids—antioxidants that mop up artery-clogging, naturally occurring chemicals in the body—may help reduce heart disease by improving the function of the endothelial cells in the arteries. To reap the rewards, choose up to two ounces of dark chocolate with a high cocoa content (70 percent or higher) each day.

In 1977, while at UC, Berkeley, doing her dietetic internship rotation at a local hospital, Birsinger and the other dietetic students were told by the chief dietitian that she had started to see cases, mostly of girls, who wouldn't eat (signs of anorexia nervosa), and if they did they would eat and then throw up the food (the bingeing and purging syndrome of bulimia nervosa). "It was the first time I ever heard that others had my problem," Birsinger told me. "But what the chief dietitian was describing did more harm than good. Talking about the psychological profile of people with eating disorders, she described them as emotional cripples, as people who have huge issues with their overcontrolling mothers, and as people with low morals who lie and steal and can't be trusted. I remember feeling frozen and thinking that I can never ever tell anybody about this. Although I now know there is a diagnosis for what I was experiencing, neither health professionals, nor I, knew what it was at the time. I decided that I could not get help from my professional or medical community because they may have this misperception and misunderstanding about me and my eating problem. Not identifying with what my teacher was saying, and feeling that nobody would understand, I went underground and decided that I had to manage my eating issues myself. But they only got worse"—until she put a permanent break on them ten years later. "I was extremely lucky I was able to do this," Birsinger explains. "Because there is so much support and professional help today that would have eased much of my loneliness and pain, I wouldn't recommend that anyone struggling with eating issues try to solve them on their own. If help for my eating disorder had been available, it would have sped my recovery."[7]

Since then, Birsinger has turned her recovery program into a teaching tool that has helped many others. Birsinger was so convinced her method could help the millions of us who medicate our emotions with food that she did her doctoral dissertation on her method.[8] And her personal experience of recovery through *intuitive eating*—knowing without conscious reasoning when to eat, what to eat, and how much to eat, and what's optimal for that individual at any given time—would serve as a model for her research.

Birsinger's Decoding Emotional Eating Program

The truly fascinating aspect of emotional eating, of course, is that not all women and men succumb to feeding their emotions with food. Those who don't use food tend to replace the urge to splurge with dealing directly with their emotions. This idea of meeting our emotional needs head on, instead of indirectly and symbolically through food, is exactly what intrigued Birsinger. Putting this insight into action had worked effectively for her, so much so that it empowered her to end her emotional eating disorder.

Those who have looked into the causes of overeating and the reasons most of us fail at dieting all agree that emotional factors play a large role. Emotional eating is such a powerful internal demon that it overrides knowledge about what to eat and tyrannizes weight loss plans. Aware of this when she began her study, Birsinger set out to do more than measure emotional eating: she was determined to develop a way to give people the skills they need to transform, and take control of, their emotional eating urges. Her core belief: if emotional as well as physical, spiritual, and social needs could be filled directly, participants would be less likely to turn to food to cope, and managing eating and weight more effectively would be a side effect of her intervention. Other key considerations: Without following a prescribed diet, can adults self-regulate their eating using intuitive tools? Can they learn to rely on their internal resources to improve their eating habits? Can they get the appropriate amount of calories and nutrients in their food, relying on their own internal resources and mind-body to eat optimally?

It was time to find out.

To tease out the answers to her questions, Birsinger took a refreshingly novel approach, a comprehensive one that considers the full spectrum of emotional, spiritual, and social factors that contribute to overeating, overweight, and obesity; she all but ignored the more typical mono-focus on *what* to eat and its straitjacket of traditional dietary recommendations. Instead, she evaluated the effectiveness of an integrative healing approach to resolve disordered eating and weight issues. To do this evaluation, she randomly assigned 102 adult women, ages 19 to 76 (median age: 51), to an intervention or control (waitlist) group: 54 healthy adult women, interested in an alternative approach to eating and weight management, were in the intuitive eating group; the 48 participants in the delayed treatment group would eat what was normal for them during the study, then they would be trained in the intuitive eating method afterward.

When the study started, each group filled out preintervention questionnaires; after the eight-week program, they filled out the same questionnaires so that changes, if any, could be measured. What is especially amazing and telling about the questionnaires she used in her study is that they not only measured eating behaviors, but they also looked at the more subtle emotional, spiritual, and social reasons that motivate people to overeat. For instance, like Eskimos who have many names for snow, Birsinger analyzed the many varieties of internal and external factors that prompt us to eat. Consider intrinsic eating (eating in response to being bored, upset, anxious, depressed, or frustrated), extrinsic eating (eating in response to food that tastes good, or when you smell something delicious), and restrained eating (intentionally consuming fewer calories than your body needs). Interestingly, Birsinger measured restrained eating by asking respondents whether their eating is restrained when their weight is up. Another aspect of the more subtle nuances Birsinger explored was about the feelings that certain foods represent to each participant.

And then the eight-week intervention began. During this time, the intervention group received sixteen hours of experiential instruction and training designed by Birsinger. Topics included intuitive eating techniques (learning to identify the difference between physical hunger and *symbolic* hunger, the desire to eat without physical hunger); decoding of symbolic food cravings; mindfulness and nonjudgmental eating; abundance, consciousness, and environmental planning for optimal foods; practicing presence; joy of movement; self- and body-acceptance; and the influence of the feminine and masculine archetypal energies on food and body issues.

To communicate the content of the intervention, Birsinger used a rich repository of teaching tools that included lectures and presentations; group, dyad, and triad discussions; question and answer sessions; guided imagery; journal exercises; right brain writing and drawing; expressive art and somatic movement activities; psychodrama/role play; meditation and contemplative practice; myths, metaphors, storytelling; and the Inner Counselor and Symbolic Visualization Process. Clearly, Birsinger's teaching methods were as diverse as the program she created, and the intervention was intensively interactive. Was the effort worth it? Did participants obtain the benefits both Birsinger and they were hoping would manifest?

The results were, in large part, what Birsinger hoped to achieve. After learning Birsinger's techniques, participants were able both to maintain their weight and to prevent gaining it back. Indeed, those who lost the most weight made the most changes in emotional eating, which suggests that overcoming this eating behavior is key if a person who struggles with weight is to be successful at overcoming emotional eating.

Birsinger's findings, though, reach far beyond weight because those who received Birsinger's intensive, extensive, and comprehensive training in intuitive and integrative practices decreased their symbolic food cravings (eating for reasons other than hunger) and overeating behaviors. And there were other beneficial outcomes: fewer compulsive eating and dieting behaviors, less anxiety about eating, and a stronger sense of connection. Attitudes toward eating improved, as did acceptance of body image, self-esteem, spiritual well-being, and self-care practices (physical activity, emotional support, etc.).[9]

Such encouraging results suggest that ongoing weight loss success hinges on changing the whole matrix of physical, emotional, spiritual, and social factors involved in overeating, overweight, and obesity. If you recall, in chapter 1, we discussed our Whole Person Nutrition Model and Program (eating for physical, emotional, spiritual, and social well-being), the essence of which is overcoming the seven eating styles, as *the* key to achieving and maintaining optimal weight and well-being. Birsinger's findings support our eating style research and its link to multidimensional well-being. Clearly, more similar studies need to be done to see whether those who participated in Birsinger's program can maintain their improved relationship to food. The more important take-away message, though, is that a whole person nutrition approach to food and eating, one that targets the multidimensional disruptive emotions that drive us to overeat, seems to be a more useful strategy than focusing on just one eating style, such as food fretting, when it comes to providing a possible solution to the obesity epidemic (pandemic?) to which so many Americans contribute.

Transformation Strategies

Right now, you're at a turning point. You can decide to take care of your physical and symbolic hunger needs for food in an appropriate way. Or you can continue to turn to food to do the job. By choosing the path of transformation, though, you're deciding to feed your body, mind, and soul what they really need; in other words, you're giving yourself true nourishment. The following exercises may not resolve all your eating problems overnight, but they can be a helpful step toward resolving your emotional eating issue if you practice them each time the urge to splurge surfaces. The secret? Birsinger's "decoding process" shows you how to shed light on unmet intrinsic needs you may have that are rooted in disordered eating. And then, symbolically, she'll show you how to transform your craving by filling your needs with something other than food.

Birsinger has a clear and strong conviction that there's a reason and a purpose for overeating. You're trying to take care of yourself on some level, to fill a need that's not getting cared for in another way. Food is available. It can do the job well, but it's only temporary—and there are side effects and consequences. If no effective self-care mechanisms are in place, your emotional eating isn't going to go away. The antidote? Develop the capacity to tolerate a range of unpleasant emotions. Birsinger offers the following two strategies for dealing with emotional eating: one for *physical* hunger; one for *symbolic* hunger.

Is Your Hunger Physical or Symbolic?

Overcoming overeating starts with discerning physical hunger from symbolic hunger. When you think of eating, is your desire to eat coming from physical hunger (located in your stomach) or symbolic hunger (eating for reasons other than for physical nourishment)? Check in now. Physical hunger is often experienced in the stomach, while symbolic hunger often manifests in the chest, throat, or mouth. In other words, *where* you're feeling the feeling is a clue about whether the hunger is physical or symbolic.

Physical hunger. *How hungry are you?* Imagine the following scenario: You're at your desk and you begin to think about eating. Ask yourself whether you're physically hungry in your body, or whether you have symbolic hunger. You realize you're actually hungry. Sitting at your desk and thinking of food is your cue to check in with your hunger level. On a scale of 1 to 10, identify your hunger level (1 is famished, 5 is neutral, at 10, you are way overfed). You identify that you're at level 3, which means you're identifying that you're physically hungry and you need to eat.

Decide what to eat and how much. Now, decide what you want to eat. How much of it do you want? To know what your mind-body wants to eat, develop a mind-body connection. You can do this by checking in with your body before eating. To begin, ask your body what it wants. Doing this, Birsinger claims, means eating from the neck *down,* instead of the neck *up* (all in your mind)—which is where most people make decisions about what to eat.

Do the guided imagery visualization. Birsinger developed the guided imagery visualization exercise on the next page to give you the skills you need to make the mind-body connection, which in turn can empower you to dramatically change what and how you eat forever. Practice it every time before you eat.

Symbolic hunger. Imagine the following scenario: You're at your desk and you begin to think about eating. Ask yourself whether you're physically hungry in your body, or whether you have symbolic hunger. Okay, you're feeling anxious, you realize. No. You're not hungry. Your hunger is symbolic, not literal and physical. You really want chocolate chip cookies to help you cope with uncomfortable emotions. Even though you're not hungry, you're still wanting to eat. What's going on? You can't wait until you're hungry. If you can wait, great. Many can't wait, though, because emotional eating is an ingrained habit. If so . . .

Birsinger suggests that you go to step 2 of the Guided Imagery Visualization Exercise. If you can have anything you want, what would it be? The intensity of the emotion will determine whether you can

Guided Imagery Visualization Exercise

1. Inhale deeply, pause for two seconds, and exhale deeply, bringing your awareness from your head to your body. Notice air moving through your lungs. Notice the movement of your stomach expanding and contracting.

2. Imagine that you could have anything on the planet to eat right now—without any judgment about the food's calorie, protein, or carbohydrate content. What would that be? No one needs to know. It's a private fantasy.

3. Now think of the amount you would love to have of this food. Again, don't bring judgment to your decision. How much would you really like to have? Imagine you can see the food and the amount you just visualized. It's just there in front of you. Is it in a serving dish? On a plate?

4. Now, you've eaten the food. Imagine this food is now in your stomach. How does it feel? Does the amount feel just right? Too much? Is it pushing on your stomach? Is it making you feel bloated? Does your stomach hurt?

5. Ask your body how much would be okay to eat so you feel comfortably full, alert, and energized.

6. Now imagine this food is moving down into your digestive system. Ask your body how the food feels in your digestive tract. Is there any discomfort in that part of your body as the food is being digested, such as pain, bloating, or gas?

7. Ask your body how much of this food would be okay to eat for you to feel good. Then, modify the amount

> you ate to fit the "feel good" amount, meaning, any
> symptoms of discomfort are gone.
> 8. Now imagine the food has been digested. The
>   nutrients are being absorbed into your bloodstream,
>   and they're circulating through the brain, through
>   the muscles, the organs, the skin; all your cell
>   tissues are now being nourished.
> 9. After envisioning the optimal amount of food you
>   can eat and still feel comfortable, scan your body
>   to see whether there are any changes in sensations
>   or feelings.

wait or not. If nothing else will help, you may need to eat that cookie. Keep in mind, though, that by doing this process before you eat, you're becoming conscious of your needs and eating behaviors—without judgment. And such nonjudgmental awareness is a key step that can diminish overeating.

Give Yourself Permission to Eat

Whether your hunger is physical or symbolic, if you really want to eat a cookie, that's what you ought to do: eat the cookie without judging yourself. A key reason people overeat is that they impose restrictions on themselves about what they should or shouldn't eat and then they don't eat what they really want. When you do this, though, you continue to "chase" whatever you were trying to get from the cookie.

Birsinger believes you won't overeat if you practice the above mind-body visualization "because we're born with this ability to 'know' what and how much to eat," she says, and the guided imagery technique, above, is a way to reconnect to this. In a way, it's like programming a computer: once you have the amount that feels good in your body, it doesn't matter how food is put in front of you. For instance, let's say you want a banana split, with whipped cream and hot fudge. But when you do this exercise, you realize the entire banana split is way too much for you to eat if you're to continue to feel comfortable in your body. When this happens, before eating, decide on the amount that'll feel good in your body, which may be only a couple of bites. Or not.

Birsinger offers this insight: If you don't do the guided imagery visualization (above), you're more likely to sit down and eat the whole banana split; you'll overeat and then feel stuffed. Self-sabotage may take over: "Now I've really blown it. That was way too much," you might think, but this only leads to more eating later because you're likely to eat to berate yourself. And then, to feel better, you're going to have to eat again, and then restrict yourself, and then exercise, and then, on the rebound, overeat again, and so on . . . Birsinger says that "all this happens because you've lost touch with your internal cues of what, when, and how much to eat. But when you make the connection to how much you need to feel okay, your mind-body remembers it. And then you—not food—are in charge of your emotions."

Transform the Craving

Here's another technique Birsinger created to help you transform negative, unpleasant feelings that lead to emotional eating, into pleasant, sense-filled emotions that fill you without food:

- Using all your senses, find ways to evoke the sense you get doing an enjoyable activity (such as yoga or meditation or taking a walk). Have a symbol nearby of something that represents the pleasurable activity, for example, a picture of a beautiful seascape, a heart-shaped paper weight, a lucky coin. Choose anything you like as a symbol that represents the activity.

- What do you love about the particular activity? For instance, if it's a walk on the beach, do you love the sound of the ocean? The air? Putting your feet in the sand?

- Find a fragrance you love. Cinnamon? Vanilla? Musk?
  To transform the craving, inhale your favorite scent. By
  doing this, you're symbolically filling up your senses with
  your favorite activity. Along with scents, you can try this
  with textures, sounds, and so on.

The key concept: Fill your senses as much as possible with the
scent until you can evoke the feeling you get when you're actually doing
your favorite activity of choice. Enjoy the journey instead of food.[10]

Fine-Tune Feelings with Food

There's another way you can take charge of emotional eating. Replace
unpleasant feelings that drive you to overeat with conscious food
choices that hold the power to enhance your mood. The following
scenario will give you an idea about how you can fine-tune your feelings to your advantage.[11]

Susan is often overwhelmed with all-day fatigue, minimal motivation, and a sluggish metabolism. Her sister, Allison, feels edgy,
irritable, and nervous, symptoms that worsen because of bouts of
indigestion that make it hard for her to fall or stay asleep. Their dad,
Tom, who has always been a competent accountant, more and more
has frequent memory lapses and trouble recalling information. Their
mom is dealing with the same old symptoms: constant cravings for
carbohydrates, feeling blue and bloated, and depressed about her
stubborn weight gain.

Be balanced. Ann, Allison, and their parents are unaware that
natural "chemical messengers" (neurotransmitters discussed earlier in
the chapter) released from foods they choose can modify their moods,
alleviate anxiety, bolster brain power—even curb the urge to splurge
on that donut—so they continue to consume their "routine cuisine."
They are not alone in their ignorance of four key neurotransmitters—
dopamine, acetylcholine, gamma-aminobutyric acid (GABA), and *serotonin*—

that influence everything from energy and mood to memory and metabolism. When these four hormones are in balance, your mind-body is poised for peak performance. But when one or more dip and cause an imbalance, symptoms ranging from fatigue and weight gain to confusion and depression can manifest. The good news: you can choose "designer foods" that reduce unpleasant feelings and unwelcome behaviors.

Enhance energy. Have you ever felt fatigue or lethargy throughout the day, even after a full night's sleep? If low energy is typical for you, the cause could be dopamine deficiency. From fabulous flavors to sensual scents, if your brain interprets a food (or an activity) as pleasurable, and you tend to turn to it for a pleasure hit, it may be because you're seeking the feel-good response of dopamine. In essence, dopamine works its wonders by stimulating the central nervous system (CNS), keeping energy levels, motivation, and excitement high.

Dopamine Rx. The pleasure-producing ingredients in high-protein foods are the amino acids *tyrosine* and *phenylalanine*, building blocks of both protein and dopamine. To elevate mood and energy, consider consuming water-packed tuna, low-fat yogurt, or lean meat.

Alleviate anxiety. If anxiety, nervousness, and irritability—with bouts of indigestion and trouble sleeping—are all too familiar symptoms, it may mean you have low levels of GABA. A nerve chemical and nerve modulator that stimulates the central nervous system, this natural sedative works its wonders by controlling brainwave rhythms, which in turn regulate behavior.

GABA Rx. Take action to produce more GABA by choosing foods high in the B vitamins, especially B_6. Although the mechanism of how B_6 affects the nervous system and brain isn't completely understood, even marginal intakes influence levels of GABA (and other mood-modifying neurotransmitters). Boost dietary intake of this B vitamin with *whole* grains, dark leafy greens, bananas, avocados, and protein-rich chicken, fish, legumes, and nuts.

Defog. Some older people call it a "senior moment"; others who find it harder and harder to recall information might say they're experiencing a memory lapse. Those who study food and mood may interpret such symptoms of "brain fog" to be a sign of acetylcholine deficiency. Produced in the brain by the fatlike substance *choline*, this nerve chemical is a building block of *myelin*, which helps CNS cells communicate.

Acetylcholine Rx. To manage general mental functioning, boost brain levels of this memory manager by consuming choline-rich foods, such as wheat germ, fish, eggs, blueberries, and peanuts, all of which are converted into acetylcholine during digestion.

Curtail cravings. Do you crave high-carbohydrate, high-salt foods, such as cookies, cake, and chips—especially when you're feeling blue? Do you feel hungry even when you're full? Is weight gain a constant? If so, your supply of serotonin may be low. Soothing serotonin is a natural antidepressant; it also contributes to stable blood sugar levels, which in turn prevents food cravings and the urge to overeat.

Serotonin Rx. To produce more serotonin, seek out foods rich in the amino acid *tryptophan*, such as avocado, poultry, and wheat germ. Other options include foods high in complex carbohydrates, such as potatoes (with the skin), beans, and whole grains.

Instead of feeding that drive to overeat, food can serve as your anti–emotional eating ally with its power to bring emotional balance, enhance your energy, alleviate anxiety, and contribute to clearer thinking. Instead of caving into cravings, put yourself in the driver's seat and take your feelings where you want them to go.

"B" Wise

From dreary doldrums to a deeper depression, various B vitamins, including B_1, B_2, niacin, folic acid, and B_{12}, can help you bust the blues. To help defeat depression, "B" wise, and consider the following guidelines when deciding which foods to eat.

Choose whole foods. Fast food "is a loser when it comes to vitamins and minerals that help to boost spirit," writes nutritionist Elizabeth Somer. Indeed, folic acid, in particular (the most common nutritional deficiency in the United states), is linked to depression, as are other B-family relatives that are processed out of refined foods: B_6, niacin, and B_{12}. Some especially good vitamin B–abundant blues busters are unprocessed, unrefined grains (whole wheat, oats, millet, brown rice, etc.), fruits, vegetables, beans, nuts, and seeds. Vitamin B–rich greens, such as spinach, are especially good blues busters.

Shake the sugar habit. When you consume a lot of refined white sugar, it both damages and destroys B vitamins in the body; in this way, it contributes to deficiencies. Eliminate sugar from the diet and depression often lifts—although why this is so is not well understood. One theory is that the high derived from sugar is due to elevated glucose (blood sugar) and endorphins, which produce feelings of relaxation and euphoria. When the sugar in food is metabolized, blood sugar levels and endorphins and other hormones "crash," contributing to depression and fatigue. When a diet is rich in foods loaded with vitamin B, and low in sugar, levels of B vitamins, glucose, and endorphins remain stable, reducing the odds of depression.

Avoid or limit alcohol and caffeine. Consuming too much alcohol and caffeine can cause the loss of certain B vitamins. And deficiencies of vitamins B_6 and niacin, especially, can bring you down. Not only does excessive alcohol and caffeine consumption reduce the absorption of B vitamins, but it also contributes to protein and mineral deficiencies.[12]

Many of us have felt sad or have had the Monday morning blahs at times; still others—more than fifteen million Americans—experience serious depression during their lifetime. Include more foods high in the B vitamins, and you may improve your mood and lower the odds of depression linked to emotional eating.

Overcoming Emotional Eating

The science that studies nutrients in the foods we consume, and the way in which they influence our brain chemistry and emotions, provides a peek into how food and the mind and body work together. By being aware of this connection, each food you choose to eat may be looked at as an opportunity not only to feed your body but also to fine-tune your moods and emotions. At the same time, the key to Enlightened Diet success is making a commitment to eat only for pleasure and when you're feeling feel-good feelings. While this chapter highlighted foods that calm and soothe and alleviate anxiety, the next chapter, on the fast foodism eating style, will give you the practical tools you need to undiet, and instead to live a food-filled life that leads to optimal, normal eating and weight, as well as to vitality, health, and well-being.

Chapter 5

Fast Foodism

$R_x:$ Choose fresh whole food in its natural state as often as possible.

One evening after physician Mark A. Hyman had given a lecture, a sixty-year-old morbidly obese man named Samuel approached him. Weighing more than three hundred pounds, Samuel asked Hyman if he would be his doctor, and Hyman agreed. During the office visit, Samuel described a life filled with excessive overeating and bingeing; for instance, two cups of heavy whipping cream each night was a typical night cap. In an attempt to lose weight, he had a history of extreme yo-yo dieting: losing weight and then gaining it back . . . and more. As his obesity worsened, so, too, did its effect on his health. By the time Samuel saw Hyman, he had a plethora of infirmities, ranging from profound fatigue, difficulty breathing while walking, stuffed sinuses, swollen legs, severe sleep apnea, dry skin, imbalanced hormones, food sensitivities, and an impaired liver, as well as a wide range of risk factors linked to heart disease, such as diabetes.

What happened next changed Samuel's health and weight, indeed his life, forever. Hyman gave him hope. "I told him that if he did everything I suggested, he would lose weight, feel better, and his symptoms would go away. Everything he had done, he did to himself and could undo," writes Hyman. What did Hyman suggest? The core of the program he recommended for Samuel was a diet abundant in nutrient-dense, fresh, unprocessed, whole foods (fruits, vegetables, whole grains, beans and peas, and nuts and seeds) "without any restriction on calories or portion size." To enhance Samuel's weight loss, Hyman included a conservative exercise plan of walking slowly, then he added interval training once Samuel was in better shape. He also augmented Samuel's fresh food diet and exercise plan with supplements and herbs that would be helpful in turning around Samuel's various ailments.

Armed with this advice, Samuel left Hyman's office somewhat skeptical but determined. After three months on the program, Samuel lost thirty pounds, his food cravings disappeared, and some of his symptoms were less severe. Eight months later, "I was shocked when he weighed in," writes Hyman. "He had lost one hundred and ten pounds without being on a strict deprivation diet." There was more good news: along with his excess weight, most of Samuel's ailments had vanished or diminished. And, just as encouraging, having replaced a diet of mostly fast, processed, fat-filled food with fresh, whole, flavor-filled nourishment, what remained was his "continued pleasure in food," writes Hyman. What is especially telling about this success story is that Samuel achieved weight and health success—without deprivation, without restricting calories, and without suffering—in large part because he replaced a predominantly high-calorie, empty-calorie, fast-food diet with a low-fat, nutrient-dense, fresh, and whole food way of eating that provided the nutrients—in the ratio nature intended—that his body needed to heal.[1]

What was it about Samuel's change from fast food to a fresh whole food way of eating that led to such powerful—seemingly effortless—improvements in his weight and well-being? And if it worked for him, might it be beneficial for the millions of us who struggle with the perennial weight loss question: what's the best diet for losing weight and keeping it off? A look at the fast foodism eating style can give us clues to ways in which a mostly fast and processed food diet increases the odds you'll be overweight and, in contrast, how consuming mostly fresh whole foods, as Samuel did, can lead to weight loss that is often effortless.

Foodish Food

Some say it's "snack crack"; others imply it's an "industrial artifact"; corporations call it a "commodity"; my friend and colleague, naturopathic physician Bruce Milliman, calls it "ersatz food," meaning "an inferior substitute imitating an original"; the Center for Science in the Public Interest (CSPI) calls it "food porn"; I call it "foodish food"—which is the opposite of the fresh, whole, lean food that helped Samuel lose weight.

Foodish food has three attributes: it is typically fast, processed, and unhealthy. Most of you are familiar with fast food, which is inexpensive and prepared and served quickly in fast food restaurants, such as McDonald's, Burger King, Wendy's, Kentucky Fried Chicken, and Taco Bell.[2] Processed food, on the other hand, has been cooked, baked, cured, heated, dried, mixed, ground, separated, extracted, sliced, preserved, dehydrated, frozen; because processed food is often manufactured, it typically includes packaging, canning, jarring, or enclosing the processed food in some other sort of container.[3] Both fast and processed foods have one thing in common: they are junk food, a slang term that refers to fare that is typically high in calories, salt, sugar, fat, and additives, and low in nutritional value, such as fiber, vitamins, and minerals;[4] hence the term "empty calories" to suggest the lack of nutrients.

Foodish food—open the newspaper on any given day and you're likely to find it reviled as the scourge of the twenty-first century. As I write, I am scanning the following headlines: "It's a Fat, Fat, Fat, Fat World: America's Blueprint for Poor Eating Is Being Spread around the Planet"; "Junk-Food Makers Face FTC Scrutiny: With Childhood Obesity Rates Rising, a Group of Food Companies Could Be Forced to Disclose Details on Marketing to Feds"; and "Sugar Coated: We're drowning in high fructose corn syrup: Do the risks go beyond our waistline?"[5]

What does the fast foodism eating style look like? A breakfast bar for breakfast; Chicken McNuggets with a Coke for lunch; and perhaps a pepperoni and sausage pizza, delivered from your nearby pizza parlor, for dinner. Add several bottles of soft drinks sipped throughout the day and some snacks of chips, cake, or cookies, and you have a profile of the fast food cuisine that is typical for many Americans. Not surprisingly, this eating style is strongly linked with overeating, overweight, and obesity. And if you're a "fast fooder," you're at increased risk for heart disease, diabetes, high blood pressure, certain cancers, and other ailments, meaning that fast foodism threatens more than your waistline.

Toxic Food Environment

Kelly Brownell, a professor of psychology, epidemiology, and public health at Yale University in New Haven, Connecticut, is a leading obesity expert. And he links the obesity epidemic in America, in large part, to the "toxic food environment" that the fast food industry has created. According to Brownell, this ranges from easy access to food-ish foods to an excess of fast food advertising. "We take Joe Camel off the billboard because it is marketing bad products to our children, but Ronald McDonald is considered cute. How different are they in their impact?" asks Brownell, meaning both cigarette smoking and consuming an excess of fast foods are health threats.[6] Add the super-sizing of servings to such fast food staples as burgers, franks, fries, fried chicken, chips, and other snack foods that are already high-calorie and superprocessed, foods that often are laden with added ingredients of health-robbing trans fats, sugar, and refined flour, and you have a fast food recipe for an alarming increase in obesity.

With Americans spending 40 percent of their food budget on restaurant meals, compared to 25 percent in 1970, many are indeed living the fast foodism eating style that is contributing to our growing girth. If you typically consume fast food that is processed, and fried or sweet, then the fast foodism eating style is a key contributor to your being overweight. A closer look at the weight-boosting ingredients that are often added to fast foods will give you a better understanding about why I believe that fast food isn't food in the classic, traditional sense of the word; rather, it is foodish food, ersatz sort-of-like-food food, but not real food—and why the modifications that make fast food, well, fast food, can contribute to your growing girth.

Take-Aways, Add-Ins

The health-robbing problem with fast food is twofold: what fast food manufacturers process out of food, and what they add. Here are the key concepts you'll need to understand what is taken out of fast food and what is added to it, and how both contribute to weight gain and threaten your health.

Take-aways. In the 1750s in England, the invention of machinery used in manufacturing changed the way we make food forever. It was the roller mill, especially—huge cylinders that could crush and separate the wheat kernel into its elements of flour, germ, and bran—that made the difference. More than a century later, porcelain mills enabled manufacturers to make white flour—in lieu of whole-wheat flour—inexpensively; ergo, white flour became a popular, easily available staple for the masses. At the time, it was called "separated food" because the mill separated the bran, germ, and endosperm (flour) elements of the whole wheat kernel. Today, we call white flour "refined" or "processed" because the white flour and health-enhancing "good" fats, vitamins, minerals, antioxidants (that protect body cells from the damaging effects of oxidation), and phytochemicals (naturally occurring substances in plant-based foods that have beneficial health effects) have been processed out of the whole kernel; white flour has also been "refined" so that it will have a long shelf life and at the same time be easy to use as a key ingredient of baked goods.

Add-ins. While wheat was being denatured, nutritional science as we know it didn't exist. Sure, in the eighteenth century French chemist Antoine-Laurent Lavoisier had defined the *calorie*, a measure of energy in food, and then in the 1840s German scientist Justus von

Leibig isolated proteins, fats, carbohydrates, and minerals in food. But these discoveries were just that—discoveries. Nothing much changed in the nutrition world until the early 1900s, when diseases of malnutrition (such as beriberi and pellagra) began to manifest throughout countries whose populations were consuming separated grains: in England and America, where white flour was popular, and in Japan and China, where the population had turned from brown rice to milled, processed, denatured white rice. To combat widespread malnutrition, food manufacturers lowered the odds of deficiency diseases by enriching (adding back to) white flour and white rice food "products" the four nutrients we knew about then (niacin, riboflavin, thiamin, and iron) that had been lost in processing. This enrichment didn't include fiber or the germ or the more than twenty-five vitamins and minerals we know about now.

Today, most of the fast food you consume that is made by the multibillion-dollar fast food industry contains more than a few added vitamins and minerals in white flour products, such as hamburger buns, bread, and pie crust. To standardize the flavor, mouthfeel, and sense of satiety of fast food, added fat and sugar have become typical ingredients of fast food fare, which increases calories. And herein lies the problem: while fast food alone isn't causing obesity rates to soar (unhealthy eating habits, lack of physical activity, or a combination of the two, and genetics and lifestyle all determine your weight; more about this in chapter 2, "Food Fretting"), in America and in country after country that adapts American eating habits—including the consumption of lots of foodish food—the prevalence of obesity increases dramatically. Consider France, for instance: childhood obesity has doubled in France in the past decade due to the adoption of American lifestyle habits, such as more fast food and less physical activity. A closer look at the weight-boosting ingredients added to fast foods gives us clues about why it puts you, and everyone who consumes a mostly fast food diet, on the fat track.

Four Fast Food Weight Boosters

From fried fish, chicken, and fries, to chips, hamburgers, tacos, and pizza, fast food served in restaurants such as McDonald's, Wendy's, Taco Bell, Denny's, and Pizza Hut are familiar to most of us. What is less known is that the food you're served from these fast food outlets is highly processed and prepared, cooked in bulk on a large scale at an industrialized central location, and then shipped to each fast food restaurant. It is during the processing procedure that a seemingly simple item, let's say, white flour–based buns, become high-calorie, high-fat, sugar-laden foodish food. And not only is lots of fat and sugar added, but the *type* of fat that's used—partially hydrogenated oil—is so toxic to your health and waistline that cities such as New York City have banned its use in restaurants. And then there are all those different types of highly processed sweeteners that wreak havoc with your weight.

Researcher Robert Lustig, professor of pediatrics at UCSF (University of California, San Francisco) Children's Hospital, describes the fast food "fat-track problem" this way: "Our current Western food environment has become highly 'insulinogenic,' as demonstrated by its increased energy density (caloric intake), high fat content, high glycemic index, increased fructose composition, [and] decreased fiber . . . ." After conducting a large-scale review (called a meta-analysis) of obesity research, Lustig concluded that too much processed fructose (a type of sugar) and not enough fiber "appear to be cornerstones of the obesity epidemic through their effects on insulin."[7]

To give you a better sense of the problematic ingredients that are *added* to fast food that pose serious health problems—ingredients that the fast food industry presents as mere ingredients—let's take a closer look at the recipe for a regular McDonald's hamburger bun. Here are the highly processed and fat-, sugar-, and calorie-rich ingredients in a McDonald's hamburger bun, listed according to quantity—from most to least:

Enriched bleached flour (bleached wheat flour, malted barley flour, thiamine, riboflavin, niacin, folic acid, reduced iron), water, high fructose corn syrup, partially hydrogenated soybean oil, yeast, contains less than 2% of each of the following: salt, calcium sulfate, calcium carbonate, calcium silicate, wheat gluten, soy flour, baking soda, emulsifier (mono- and diglycerides, diacetyl tartaric acid esters of fatty acids, ethanol, sorbitol, polysorbate 20, potassium propionate), sodium stearoyl lactylate, dough conditioner (cornstarch, ammonium chloride, ammonium sulfate, calcium peroxide, ascorbic acid, azodicarbonamide, enzymes), calcium propionate (preservative). Contains wheat and soybean ingredients.[8]

The unfamiliar ingredients in a McDonald's bun may seem daunting, but it is the three "silent killers"—white flour, high fructose corn syrup, and partially hydrogenated oil—which are abundant in the buns and many other fast foods, that warrant your attention and concern if you want weight loss and well-being.

Enriched bleached flour. As you may recall, earlier in this chapter, I mentioned that enriched flour is made by first separating the three original elements of the whole wheat kernel—the flour, germ, and bran, or outer shell. The life-giving nutrients found in the germ (which has all eight B vitamins, and naturally occurring healing substances called *phytochemicals*), and the nutrients in the bran (mostly fiber and B vitamins), as well as the fiber itself, have been removed. What's left is the white flour, the *endosperm* part of the kernel, which consists mostly of carbohydrates and protein, and an unbalanced ratio of macronutrients (fat, carbohydrates, protein) and micronutrients (vitamins and minerals). Add denatured white flour to the missing fiber you need to slow down the absorption of food in your digestive system, and you've created a formula for making and retaining fat. Consume lots of white flour food products, and your odds of gaining weight are increased, because white flour food products are absorbed quickly by your body; in turn, glucose (sugar) and insulin (a hormone or "chemical messenger") levels in your body rise, along with the amount of circulating fat.

High fructose corn syrup. "Sugar: the ingredient you can trust. And pronounce. There's just one ingredient in real, all-natural sugar: real, all-natural sugar. Plus, it's only 15 little calories per teaspoon. And that's all there is to it."[9] This ad by the sugar industry, which presents sugar as a natural ingredient that is low in calories, recently ran in my local newspaper. Is it accurate? Absolutely. At the same time, though, it hides the whole story: what's hidden is the powerful place sugar takes in the creation of fast, processed foods. Call it sugar, sucrose, fructose, maple syrup, molasses, dextrose, turbinado, amazake, sorbitol, carob powder, or high fructose corn syrup—it's sugar. Regardless of how sugar is presented in its many guises on food labels, it is added to most fast foods—and it is added abundantly.

I chose as an example of fast food a seemingly innocuous hamburger bun because, unlike a donut, most of us don't think of a bun as having a lot of sugar, fat, or calories. But it does. When I looked up the carbohydrate content (sugar is carbohydrate dense) of a McDonald's hamburger, I learned it has 37 grams of carbohydrates. Because meat doesn't have any carbohydrates (meat is composed of protein and fat and vitamins and minerals), this means that a hamburger bun, by itself, has the equivalent of more than nine teaspoons, or three tablespoons, of sugar.

If you recall, the ad I told you about earlier in this section from the sugar industry said that one teaspoon of sugar is "only 15 little calories per teaspoon. And that's all there is to it." But that's not all there is to it—not when a McDonald's hamburger bun, which is not even known for being a sweet—has more than 135 calories from sugar alone! And the fact that the sugar sweetener is in the form of high fructose corn syrup (HFCS) really raises a health alarm—as well as a notch on your belt. Here's why: When you consume the fructose (a form of sugar from fruit) in the superprocessed HFCS that is added to thousands of fast foods and beverages, such as soft drinks, your brain doesn't recognize that it's a food or that it has calories (energy), although it is, indeed, calorie dense. Instead, your brain thinks you're undereating and starving; to compensate, it signals you to keep eating. In other words, HFCS ignites your hunger signals, and though you're consuming lots of calories, you're still hungry; in response to your activated appetite, you eat more . . . and gain more weight.[10]

Partially hydrogenated oil. Unlike naturally occurring polyunsaturated, monounsaturated, and saturated fat found in food, partially hydrogenated oil is an artificial creation that industry makes from plant-based foods, such as fruit, vegetables, grains, beans and peas (legumes), and nuts and seeds. To make the health menace, food manufacturers pump hydrogen atoms into liquid oils (making them "partially hydrogenated") in order to thicken them, enhance flavor, and increase the shelf life of foods that contain partially hydrogenated oil. This process is possible because hydrogenation changes the molecular structure of the oil, which in turn decreases the oil's rancidity (decomposing and becoming stale). A perfect example of oil that has been partially saturated with hydrogen atoms and therefore thickened is liquid corn oil that has been turned into a spreadable, soft margarine, or into vegetable shortening (such as Crisco). When a food or oil is completely—rather than partially—saturated with hydrogen atoms, the result is hard, firm fat, the kind you see in chilled bacon, beef, or butter.

So what's the problem? Why have cities such as New York banned food prepared with partially hydrogenated oils in restaurants? Why has it become such a threat? The answer is that the partial hydrogenation process creates *trans fatty acids*, commonly called *trans fat*, a side effect of its industrial roots. Unlike naturally occurring polyunsaturated and monounsaturated fats in food, artificially made trans fats pose serious health risks. Whether the health threat is heart disease, type 2 diabetes, or obesity, the siren has been sounded—loudly—by health professionals nationwide, and in Canada and countries throughout Europe, against trans fats. The consensus: trans fat is not safe; if you consume foods with trans fat, keep your intake to one gram or less.[11] You can get help doing this by looking at the label. As of January 2006, trans fat is listed with saturated fat and cholesterol on the Nutrition Facts label of packaged foods.

To decrease body fat, one of the best actions you can take is to avoid any food that has partially hydrogenated oil listed as one of its ingredients because *trans fat makes you fatter than other fats do*. With 8 percent of calories coming from olive oil (which consists mostly of monounsaturated fat), and 8 percent coming from industrially made trans fat, researchers at Wake Forest University fed the same number of calories to monkeys over a six-year period. When they compared the weights of the monkeys, those who ate trans fats gained four times more weight than the monkeys who consumed the olive oil–based diet. The key fast food culprits that contain trans fat: fried and baked food products.

Calories. Denatured white flour, high fructose corn syrup, and trans fats are key players on the fast food field when it comes to putting on pounds, but *the* major player, unequivocally, is the large number of calories that are in the sugar and fat that is in the super-sized portions that are offered in our nation's 300,000 fast food restaurants. The arithmetic is easy: large portions equal large waistlines. Due to supersizing and the dense number of calories in the added sugar and fat, fast food aficionados consume about 200 calories more each day than they did a decade ago. This increase in calories may not seem like much, but it could mean that you gain as much as five pounds each year; kids can put on six pounds a year from fast food. This isn't surprising when you consider a sample meal from McDonald's: a Big Mac sandwich (7.8 ounces) has 560 calories; a medium serving of french fries (4 ounces) is 380 calories; and a medium Coca-Cola (21 ounces) comes to 210 calories. Total calories in one meal: 1150.[12]

Clearly, the predominant ingredients in fast food (denatured white flour, high fructose corn syrup, partially hydrogenated oil, and lots of calories), and Americans' love affair with this foodish food, have created a deep, multidimensional problem in the United States.

Even though a diet of mostly foodish food plays havoc with our health and weight, one-quarter of our adult population visits a fast food restaurant on any given day. We are, indeed, a fast food nation.

There is a simple way to eat that is the antidote to fast foodism. It is a time- and science-tested guideline that has nourished humankind for millennia. And it is how people who are naturally thin eat today. The secret of eating to get slim and stay slim is in four simple words: fresh, whole, lean food—the dietary advice that physician Mark Hyman gave to Samuel, his morbidly obese patient, whom I told you about earlier in the chapter. By following this general guideline, Samuel was able to lose 110 pounds without eating-by-number: calorie-counting, weight watching, and counting carbs. It worked for him, and it can work for you. And there's more good news: the foods you eat for a healthy weight are the same as those for a healthy body and mind.

Inverse Eating

You've heard it before: eat five or more serving of fruits and vegetables every day. But though Uncle Sam's latest dietary recommendations have been touted on TV and in newspapers nationwide, only about 10 percent of us manage to actually do this. Why are such seemingly simple dietary guidelines so hard for so many of us to follow? In my opinion, simply put, it's just not how most Americans eat. Rather, our daily diet more typically includes food from the animal-based food groups of dairy, poultry, meat, and fish. And not only do we eat a lot of these foods, but we also often eat them in the form of fast and processed food. Here's a sampling: dairy, such as ice cream; chicken that's been fried, such as Kentucky Fried Chicken (sometimes served abundantly in buckets); processed meat, such as salami, bacon, and ham; and canned tuna "marinated" in added oil and salt.

The other side of the food-group spectrum is the plant-based food groups that typically don't make it to the American table: fruits, vegetables, *whole* grains (such as brown rice, oats, barley, whole wheat, and the less familiar quinoa), legumes (beans and peas), and nuts and seeds. Before I tell you about the slimming secrets of plant-based foods (hint: there's more to it than fewer calories), and lean, fresh, animal-based foods, you'll get a lot more from this chapter if you know this key concept about food: fruits, vegetables, whole grains, legumes, and nuts and seeds are the only naturally occurring plant-based food groups; dairy (such as milk, cheese, and yogurt), eggs, poultry (fowl in general, for example, chickens, turkey, and duck), meat (both red meat and white meat, such as beef and pork), and fish (from tuna and salmon to sole and halibut) are the only animal-based food groups.

Most of us develop weight problems because typical American fare focuses mostly on foods that *aren't* fresh, whole, and lean; they're typically highly processed, packaged fast food that is replete with calories, health-harming fat, denatured white flour, and sugar. Examples include salami instead of lean beef; ice cream instead of a single sliver of fresh artisan cheese or some nonfat milk; fried chicken instead of grilled, lean chicken breasts; and a donut or Danish instead of multigrain cereal with no added sugar. If plant-based foods are in our diet at all, they often manifest in the form of french fries; sweets, such as cake, pie, and cookies, all made with white flour and lots of added fat and sugar; bread made with white flour and high fructose corn syrup; or a sprinkling of lettuce (usually iceberg) and tomato that we flavor with bottled dressing high in fat, sugar, and calories. In other words, we eat lots of *processed* dairy, poultry, meat, and fish, with smaller, occasional (or no) servings of denatured fruits, vegetables, grains, legumes, seeds, and roasted, salted, and fat-laden nuts (such as peanut butter with added trans fat). Clearly, fresh, whole foods are mostly missing from the menu. And often if we do choose whole grain bread, a close look at the label reveals it's laden with unwanted additives, such as HFCS or partially hydrogenated oil. With the typical American diet as a starting point, I use the term "inverse eating" to describe the *opposite* of how more and more Americans are eating. Inverse eating describes a diet that consists mostly of fresh, whole, plant-based foods that are supplemented—almost as if they were condiments—with small servings of fresh, lean, low-fat meat, poultry, fish, or dairy foods. For thousands of years, inverse eating has been the norm for most cultures—and their populations are thinner and healthier for it. Take the much-touted Mediterranean diet, for instance. The foods eaten daily by people living in countries such as Greece, Italy, Spain, and Portugal hasn't changed much in thousands of years. It still emphasizes fruits, vegetables, grains, and legumes, with low to moderate amounts of dairy, poultry, and fish. Small servings of red meat are only occasional fare, and in Greece, the fat comes mostly from fresh-pressed olive oil (meaning, it has no trans fat), feta cheese (which is naturally low-fat), and fresh yogurt.

Researchers from Cornell, Oxford, and Beijing universities were so intrigued by the inverse way of eating in China that they spent a decade studying the relationship between China's ancient diet and the health of its citizens. Called the China Project, the study began in 1983 when scientists began analyzing the diets of 6,500 families in 130 rural villages that were not yet infiltrated by Western fast food available in larger cities. The data they collected and began to analyze in 1990 confirmed a diet based on grains (in the south) and corn, wheat, and millet (in the north); mineral-dense vegetables; and protein from soybeans and grains. Meat and other animal-based foods were eaten only occasionally and as condiments—seemingly to improve or adjust its flavor—except during special banquets and feasts.

Digging further into the data, the researchers discovered that the traditional, time-tested Chinese diet consisted of 75 percent calories from carbohydrates, 10 percent from protein (mostly from plant-based food), and 15 percent from fat. What a contrast to Americans' way of eating: an average of 45 to 50 percent total calories from carbohydrates, 15 percent from protein (most of which is from animal sources), and about 35 percent from fat. While China was once considered to have one of the leanest populations worldwide, the influx of American fast food has taken its toll. Today, out of a total population of 1.3 billion, 14.7 percent (184 million) are overweight, and another 2.6 percent (31 million) are obese. Still, these numbers are relatively low compared with the United States, where about two-thirds of adults are either overweight or obese. Sadly, children are catching up with the adults, and with dire results: for the first time in American history, children are expected to have shorter longevity than their parents because of their ever-increasing weight.[13]

Such statistics are the result of fast foodism and the other eating styles in this book, and a sedentary lifestyle we were never meant to live (more about this in chapter 9, "Enlightened Exercise"). Does this sound familiar? You become what you eat. In the same way, you weigh how you live. The more you identify with each eating style, and the less you move, the more likely it is that you weigh more than is optimal for you. Your lifestyle—especially your relationship to food and eating—is a key determinant of your weight. What knowledgeable health professionals nationwide would like you to do about this is to use the incredible information we've discovered about food, nutrition, and weight over the decades to start a personal revolution, to take a stand against foodish food, and instead to make fresh, whole, lean food and inverse eating your most-of-the-time way of eating.

Please note that we use the expression "your most-of-the-time way of eating" because we're suggesting fresh, whole, lean food *as often as possible*—not as a rigid, regimented, restricted way of eating. When you choose to have fast food or any other food that isn't fresh, whole, and lean—enjoy it! Now that we've made it clear that we're not suggesting a traditional diet (chapter 2, "Food Fretting" tells you more about how dieting can actually sabotage weight loss), consider this: What if you took the fresh, whole food information you need to get and stay slim, and you actually put it into action every day? How would you feel? How would you look? How would it influence your weight?

Eat More, Weigh Less

It really is possible to eat more and weigh less.[14] Doesn't such a suggestion go against everything we've learned about weight loss? Actually, what "eat more, weigh less" really means is that if you eat more of certain *types* of food, instead of focusing on the *amount* of food you eat—like Samuel, the morbidly obese man I told you about earlier in the chapter, who lost weight following his doctor's fresh, whole food advice—you, too, are likely to lose weight. Calories from fast food, and calories from fresh, whole, lean food, are not the same. Consider this:

Fruit. An apple a day may do more than keep the doctor away; it may also keep you slim. When researchers from the State University of Rio De Janeiro in Brazil put two groups of women on a *comparable calorie diet*, those who snacked on an apple lost more weight than those who munched on oatmeal cookies. Some possible reasons: With an 85 percent water content and lots of soluble fiber, apples are filling; they also keep blood sugar levels even, which cuts cravings and signals to your brain that you're full. And because apples are fresh and whole, they supply your mind-body with the nutrients you need in the balanced ratio intended by nature.

Vegetables. Studies have linked abundant mixed salads, as well as cauliflower, with weight loss. By "abundant," I'm referring to more than the typical iceberg lettuce and tomato duo that passes for a salad for many of us; rather, I'm talking about a resplendent mix of veggies that may include mixed greens, spinach, and arugula tossed with cherry tomatoes, chopped mushrooms, sliced cucumber, chopped red and green peppers, sliced avocado, beans, lean chicken or baked tofu, a sprinkling of chopped walnuts, grated cheese, and perhaps some raisins. Not only is such a salad filling and delicious, but when researchers at Penn State University studied women who consumed a satisfying salad prior to eating a pasta lunch, they discovered that they ate less pasta than those who ate pasta only.

There are still other weight loss benefits to fruits and vegetables: vitamin C is found in fruits and vegetables only. A study from Purdue University suggests it may be a key weight loss helper, because vitamin C helps you burn fat during physical activity; in fact, the study suggests vitamin C is a key determinant of weight loss.

Whole grains. Since whole grains were cultivated more than ten thousand years ago, they have been a boon to health. Now, recent research from Harvard, published in the *Journal of Clinical Nutrition*, reveals that they also prevent weight gain. In a twelve-year study with more than twelve thousand nurses from ages thirty-eight to sixty-three, researchers found that those who ate the most whole grain foods (such as oatmeal, popcorn, wheat germ, and multigrain breakfast cereal) weighed less than those who ate the least. And the difference was quite significant: women in the high whole grain group had a 49 percent lower risk of gaining weight.

Legumes. It's a fact. Including dried beans, such as pintos, navy, and lima (not green beans or soybeans) in your diet can help you lose weight. When Maurice Bennink, professor of nutrition at Michigan State University, reviewed a plethora of studies that had been published on beans over a twenty-five-year period, he discovered a compelling wealth of evidence that beans work their weight loss wonders in three ways: satiety, because beans are rich in fiber, so you feel full; sustained energy, because beans have a very low glycemic index, and thus glucose is released slowly into the bloodstream, so your blood sugar stays stable over time; and lower odds that you'll eat calorie-dense fast foods, because consuming low glycemic index foods tends to lead to subsequent choices of low glycemic index foods.

Nuts and seeds. Although they look like nuts, taste like nuts, and crunch like nuts, technically, peanuts are a legume. Because most of us relate to them as nuts, I am telling you about the potential of *fresh, raw, unroasted* peanuts as part of an eating plan for weight management in the "nuts and seeds" category. Although I wouldn't call any kind of high-fat nut a weight loss food, large population studies have linked their consumption to lower weight than for nonconsumers.

To test these survey results, Richard Mattes and his team in the Department of Foods and Nutrition at Purdue University studied three groups, each of which consumed 500 calories of peanuts: people in group one, who ate the peanuts without any dietary directions, gained an average of only 2.2 pounds; those in the second group, who added the peanuts to their usual diets, gained only one pound; and the people in the third group, who were asked to follow a low-fat diet and to substitute 500 calories of peanuts for 500 calories from other foods, maintained their weight. The mechanism by which peanuts minimize weight gain or help us maintain weight isn't completely clear; what is theorized, though, is that peanuts may work by being super-filling.

Dairy. At least one type of dairy food has been linked with lower weight: low-fat yogurt. When researchers at the University of Tennessee in Knoxville put people on a twelve-week weight-loss program, those who consumed three servings of yogurt daily lost twice as much weight at the dieters who did not eat yogurt. The study's lead researcher, Michael B. Zemel, speculates that the metabolic reason for this is that the calcium *combined with the bio-active compounds in yogurt* speeds up the fat-burning process, while at the same time, decreases the production of fat.

Eggs. It was only a one-day study, which makes it hard to draw conclusions, but there seems to be something slimming about eggs. When researcher Nikhil Dhurandhar from Pennington Biomedical Research Center in Baton Rouge, Louisiana, first gave study participants two eggs for breakfast, and then later in the study, bagels, the two-egg breakfast eaters consumed as much as 400 fewer calories than when they had bagels for breakfast. A possible reason for the difference in calories: it's likely that high-protein, low-fat eggs promote satiety more than processed, white-flour bagels. (Note: Because eggs are high in *dietary* cholesterol, they can raise your *blood* cholesterol levels. So if you have heart disease, limit or avoid consumption of eggs.)

Fish. As with eggs, fish is high in protein and low in fat. And as with the above egg study, researchers at the Karolinska Institutet in Sweden found that when people consumed fish for lunch, in comparison to those fed a beef-based meal—with both meals containing the same number of calories—the fish eaters consumed 11 percent less for dinner. It may be the protein that's filling, or, suggests lead researcher Saeedah Borzoei, it could be the rich flavor of fish (more about the flavor of food and weight in chapter 8, "Sensory Disregard"). Interestingly, steamed white fish (such as halibut) ranks number one as the most filling food (out of thirty-eight foods) in the Australian Satiety Index.

Vitamins in fruits and vegetables. Bio-active compounds in yogurt, fiber in plant-based foods, whole grains and whole apples, fresh fish—what the fresh food groups have in common is that the components in each food add up to more than the sum of their parts. In other words, while scientists have isolated particular nutrients in food that are either health enhancing or health robbing, the key to optimal nourishment is not to pursue the "parts" of food by turning mostly to synthetic supplements for health and well-being. Rather, nature is the best nutritionist possible: *consume fresh whole foods in their natural state as often as possible,* and you'll be obtaining nutrients in the ratio nature intended; in turn, your mind and body are given the nutrients they need to be balanced and healthier. Why is this so? The many ingredients in fresh, whole, lean foods—many we know about, and many more that remain to be discovered—not only balance your weight and keep you lean, but they also help prevent, treat, and reverse a plethora of ailments, from heart disease and diabetes to high blood pressure, cataracts, and arthritis. In other words, you receive many, many benefits when you inversely consume food that is as close to its natural state as possible because fresh whole fruit, vegetables, grains, legumes, and nuts and seeds, low- or nonfat dairy, and lean fish, poultry, and meat, have the whole package of nutrients for optimal health and well-being.[15]

Overcoming Fast Foodism

Throughout this chapter, we've introduced you to the ways in which foodish food can make you fat and, in contrast, how choosing fresh whole foods in their natural state as often as possible can lead to leanness—as well as to a lifetime of delicious dining. Consuming fresh whole foods can also be antidotes to the other eating styles; for instance, it is truly satisfying, so you're less likely to overeat; it contains nutrients that enhance emotions; and it is flavor filled, making it easier to eat mindfully. In the next chapter, "Solo Dining," we give you insights into the rewards of sharing food—especially fresh, tasty food, prepared with regard—with others. We are excited to be telling you about the eating style of solo dining because not only does it show you how to turn dining with others into a balm for body, heart, and soul (remember, the Enlightened Diet is a whole person nutrition and eating program that includes thriving through social support while dining), but it also reveals how eating with others more often than not helps heal what writer Elizabeth Cady Stanton described as "the solitude of self."

Chapter 6

Solo Dining

Ŗ : Share food-related experiences
with others.

One of my most memorable meals wasn't an actual meal; it was a dining experience cradled in hospitality, friendship, and fresh, simple food. The place: the patio of a friend's villa in a medieval town in Switzerland. The time: nearing midnight. The setting: like a Turner painting, an almost-full moon lighting the nearby lake. The food: an assortment of Italian cheeses, apples and oranges, and rich red wine. The social ingredients: my husband, Larry; friends; and Frau Bucher, our hostess. As the evening evolved, so too did my sense of satisfaction, for each person made a spontaneous toast at intervals throughout the evening that linked our hearts and souls and flavored the food—indeed, the entire evening—with love. Since then, I've thought often about how I might imbue my meals with the same soul-satisfying ambiance that permeated that evening. Somehow, the thought wouldn't let go.

Perhaps it was divine intervention. Or fate. Or similar sensibilities. I was gifted with the answer to my quest one New Year's Eve when I met Nailia Menne at our friend Roslyn Layton's home. Originally from Kazakhstan, Nailia told me about the *tamada* tradition when I mentioned that the English language needed a new word to describe the invisible ingredients that created the "meal magic" I had experienced that moonlit night in Switzerland. "There is an ancient tradition that no Kazakh celebration is complete without wine and a *tamada*, the host or toastmaster whose role is to create a pleasurable ambiance and ensure that everyone present is honored and enjoys the occasion," Nailia told me. "Whether the gathering is small or is a meal for many, it is a great honor for the person who is asked to be the *tamada*. Throughout the meal, starting with the elderly for whom there is much respect, followed by those who have traveled far for the occasion, the *tamada* invites each guest to toast people, the food, or the event. From the first course to the main course and then dessert, the *tamada* invites a toast," Nailia continued. "In this way, every person is honored through the modern expression of an ancient tradition that embodies the best of friendship and shared food."

As New Year's Eve continued to unfold, I knew I had found not only the word but also a time-honored ritual that embodies the special spirit of that moonlit evening in Switzerland. And now I would like to make a toast: this chapter is dedicated to *tamada*-flavored food and friendship . . . for everyone . . . all ways, all days.

Fare for One

We are a lonely culture, and nowhere is this more evident than in the millions who eat meals alone. While a *tamada*-flavored meal includes food and friendship and a welcoming and memorable dining experience for all, more often than not, an eat-alone dining scene plays out daily for millions of Americans: children reach for a piece of packaged pizza, then eat it at the computer; single working women heat up their low-cal frozen meal in the microwave, then dine solo while watching TV; or anxious traveling salesmen are driven to dashboard dining in their cars while en route to yet another meeting. Not surprisingly, these scenarios also reflect the other eating styles: food fretting, task snacking, emotional eating, fast foodism, unappetizing atmosphere, and sensory disregard. This phenomenon isn't surprising; after all, the eating styles are an interconnected, related family of eating choices and behaviors that lead to overweight and obesity.

Not only does our research shed light on the social isolation that surrounds food and dining, but it also links eating alone more often than not with an increased likelihood of being overweight or obese. Indeed, our research on the eating styles revealed that the more often people dine alone, the higher their body mass index (BMI), which is the measure for weight levels. In contrast, we found that normal weight people typically eat with others and that they are also more likely to eat wholesome fresh food and less fast, processed, and pre-pared food (see chapter 5, "Fast Foodism," for more about this weight-inducing eating style). This observation is a sobering fact because it suggests that chronic social isolation while dining increases the odds that not only will you overeat but also that you'll eat more of the kinds of food that can easily add pounds.

There is yet another way to make sense of solo dining: children, t'weens, and teens who don't eat dinner with other family members, such as siblings and parents, are at high risk for supersizing them-selves. The problem of solo dining and its link to increased risk of various health problems has so invaded our culture that Joseph A. Califano Jr., chairman and president of the National Center on Addic-tion and Substance Abuse at Columbia University and former secre-tary of the Department of Health, Education, and Welfare, has initiated "Family Day—A Day to Eat Dinner with Your Children."[1] For those of you who think that addiction and substance abuse have nothing to do with food and overeating, consider this: millions of Americans who overeat and zone out with fast food, do, indeed, have a substance abuse problem; while they may not literally be addicted to food, they have a strong physiological or psychological dependency on food and a habit of overeating, which ultimately damages their weight and self-esteem. Why are children and adolescents who don't eat meals with their families more prone to obesity? Some research-ers have put this exact question to the test.

Family Fare

When Harvard researcher Matthew Gillman looked at the eating habits of more than sixteen thousand boys and girls aged nine to fourteen, he discovered that those who usually or always ate dinner with their families were more likely to consume more fruits and vegetables, less soda, and less fried, high-fat, and sugar-laden food. And we know from our eating styles research that fast, processed foods are strong predictors of weight. Not surprisingly, Gillman's study also revealed that while 43 percent ate dinner with their families daily, the older the child, the less often he or she shared in the family meal.[2]

Richard Strauss, director of the Childhood Weight Control Program at the Robert Wood Johnson Medical School in New Brunswick, New Jersey, is another academic who warns that not getting together at dinnertime is contributing greatly to our epidemic of childhood obesity. Indeed, with one in five American kids being overweight and still more suffering from obesity, the growing girth of adolescents has become an urgent national health problem. Sure, limited physical activity plays a part—the children in Strauss's study spent only twelve minutes daily doing hard, sustained exercise; most spent up to five hours indoors playing video games and watching TV. More threatening to health, though, is that they consume typically high-fat, large portions of food and excessively sweet sodas. Merge inactivity with mostly high-calorie meals eaten outside the home and you have a recipe for a way of life that contributes to obesity and ensuing medical complications, such as hypertension, diabetes, high cholesterol, and orthopedic problems; a lifetime of low self-esteem is also often part of the teenage obesity package.

With our health and that of our children at stake, Strauss firmly believes that the solution lies in the problem. The antidote he suggests is to share family fare filled with fresh fruits, vegetables, whole grains (such as brown rice, oatmeal, and so on), legumes, and low-fat and lean dairy, fish, poultry, and meat (see chapter 5, "Fast Foodism," to learn how to create fresh family fare), and to increase physical activity together (see chapter 9, "Enlightened Exercise," for ideas on including more motion in your life). Strauss predicts, perhaps somewhat ominously, that without making fresh food and more activity a family affair, the obesity epidemic will continue.[3]

Social Ties

The idea that family meals can serve as a buffer against ailments emerged in a landmark twenty-five-year study that began in the early 1960s in the small town of Roseto, Pennsylvania, when a local physician told researcher Stewart Wolf that he rarely saw cases of heart disease in the town's Italian-American population. Intrigued, Wolf set out to study the Rosetans, hoping to discover why their rate of heart disease was so low, even though they consumed a traditionally high-fat, high-cholesterol Italian-American diet of sauces, sausages, and other artery-clogging food. Wolf was especially fascinated because the rate of heart disease and mortality from heart attacks remained low in Roseto regardless of the inhabitants' diet.

As the long-term study progressed, so too did the rate of heart disease among the Italian-Americans—so much so that it soon equaled that of the general American population. When Wolf and his colleagues scrutinized the data, the key difference that surfaced was the change in the Italian-Americans' human relationships. When the study started, close family ties and community cohesion were the norm—so much so that it was common to find three generations of Italians living together in one home. But as the children grew into adults, they moved away from Roseto. Over time, the close family ties and community cohesion began to unravel and weaken, along with commitment to religion, relationships, and traditional values. The close-knit way of life that had united Rosetans since they had migrated to America in 1882 had ended—along with its prophylactic effect on heart disease.

Although the Roseto study explores the shift in heart disease of an Italian-American community over a quarter century, it is also about the influence of human relationships and social support on the metabolism of high-fat, high-cholesterol, calorie-dense foods. Amazingly, this study suggests that when social support is present in our lives, especially when we eat, *what* we eat is somehow metabolized differently—even if that food is typically artery-clogging. If social support can halt heart disease even when we consume foods that are typically perceived as *not* being heart healthy, might family fare also influence the way in which we metabolize high-fat, calorie-dense food, and ultimately, whether we gain weight—or not?[4]

Care-Filled Feeding

With uncanny foresight, research results on the people of Roseto seemed to have anticipated future studies that would serendipitously link dining with others to health and healing benefits. Not too long after the Roseto study, researcher Robert M. Nerem also discovered that there is an invisible healing web inherent in relationships and the way in which we metabolize potentially artery-clogging food. When Nerem started his study, he set out to learn about the effect diet has on the development of coronary artery disease (CAD). To find out, a research assistant on his team fed high-cholesterol bits of rabbit chow to rabbits kept in cages. When it was time to tally the results, they were confounded because even though all the rabbits were fed the same artery-clogging food, some of them had 60 percent less plaque (blockage) in their arteries.

Unable to understand why some rabbits showed early signs of heart disease and others didn't, Nerem and his team retraced each step of the study. Again, the rabbits in the middle tier of cages fared better than those in the lower and higher rungs. Upon closer scrutiny, they discovered that it was the rabbits in the middle tiers that the research assistant would take out of their cages so that she could hold, pet, talk to, and play with as she fed them. Apparently, because it was harder for the petite assistant to reach the rabbits in the higher and lower tiers, those in the middle cages received their food while being held. Amazed, the scientists repeated the same study under much more measured conditions. This time, some rabbits would be fed the high-cholesterol diet while being individually held on a regular basis, while those in the control group would be fed the same diet and be given normal laboratory animal care, but they wouldn't be personally nurtured while being fed. Again, the cared-for rabbits showed more than a 60 percent reduction in lesions compared to the comparison group, even though the serum cholesterol levels, heart rate, and blood pressure of all the rabbits were similar.[5]

Given that both the Roseto and the rabbit experiments imply that there is a mystery to how we metabolize food, and that the consciousness we bring to meals matters, I think it is worth repeating something from the very beginning of this book, a quotation from physician Deepak Chopra describing just how powerful invisible nutrients, such as social support, can be to our health and well-being. "When you look at nutrition from a purely scientific point of view, there is no place for consciousness. And yet, consciousness could be one of the crucial determinants of the metabolism of food itself."

These studies on the power of relationships and food metabolism are amazing because they suggest that social support, and both intentional and unintentional awareness we bring to meals, impacts the way our bodies use nutrients and other substances in our food—so much so that it has the power to halt the development of heart disease. Call it awareness, realization, or perception, the "consciousness" to which Chopra alludes suggests a special sensibility or sensitivity—an invisible, hard-to-measure mystery—that somehow plays an essential and critical role in "the metabolism of food itself." And when this consciousness is miraculously activated, not only can it neutralize potentially artery-clogging cholesterol and fat we've consumed, but it also protects us against disease. Imagine! The bottom line: without drugs or surgery or following a special diet, you have the power to activate the mystery of consciousness and influence the way you metabolize food—and potentially, your waistline and health—simply by dining in the company of others.

Resetting the American Table

Even though the above studies suggest that many benefits await us when we turn a table for one into a feast for a few, eating alone is a way of life with which many of us are all too familiar. Americans are paying a big price for their often secluded, mindless munching, for what *San Francisco Chronicle* food columnist and cookbook author Marion Cunningham describes as "a motel life," meaning going in, going out, then grabbing something to eat alone. "When you eat this way, you don't create deep connections," says Cunningham, "and you miss the opportunity to get to know about the people you're living with when you don't sit around the table and share yourself around food."

In the 1970s, aware of the trend of the disappearing family meal in America, the American Institute of Wine and Food created a group called Resetting the American Table. Its mission is to alert parents to start cooking for their families. As a member of this group, national treasure Marion Cunningham, now in her eighties, feels strongly about the need for what she calls "social nourishment." Cunningham told me that "we're fed more than food when we eat with others. Instead of taking a solitary trip through life, when you dine with family you learn to share and care for others, as well as social skills, tradition, and ritual. Talk begins to flow, feelings are expressed, and a sense of well-being takes over."[6] Such is the nourishment that beckons when we reset the American table.

Recipes for Social Satisfaction

When I'm giving presentations and I'm discussing social nutrition and the solo dining eating style, I often offer the following scenario for consideration: Imagine it's wintertime at 6:30 p.m., and you're in your car, driving home from work. It's dark and cold outside, you're fairly hungry (on a 1 to 10 scale, if 1 is famished and 10 is stuffed, you're at level 3), and you won't be home for half an hour. As you drive in rush-hour traffic, not only are you hungry, but you're also feeling alone and isolated. But then you think about the meal that awaits you. You know that your grandmother, who lives with you, your spouse, and your three adolescent children, has been making dinner for you and your family for the past few hours. You know that when you enter your home, your first greeting will be the aroma of your grandmother's freshly made meal. As you hang up your coat, you'll glance at the dining table, which, as always, is set with place settings for six; sighing with delight, you'll think about how welcoming it looks, and how lucky you are to come home to a home-cooked meal with your family. As you continue driving, somehow your reverie of what awaits you has kept your hunger in check. It is no longer gnawing at you, tempting you to stop at a fast food outlet to get something—perhaps a muffin—to appease your appetite. Somehow, just the thought of the fresh, family meal has filled you enough that your hunger isn't setting off sirens of discomfort; instead, you realize that it's merely a signal that it's time for you to eat.

When I ask people to share their reaction to this family-fare scene, I often hear sighs of satisfaction, and comments such as: "I feel peaceful," "I'm envious," or "I wouldn't fear my hunger and rush to fill it with fast food." What follows are some recipes—both literal and figurative—for starting your own social nutrition traditions—and for turning a table for one into a table for two, three, or more.

Set a Friendship-Flavored Table

In ancient Rome, after a three-course meal, the host of the evening would ask guests to chose a *magister bibendi*, a toastmaster who was responsible for each person's alcohol consumption; this honored person would also select speakers for the evening and decide on topics for convivial conversation. If we take our cue from both the ancient Romans as well as the *tamada* toast made by the host throughout a meal, which I told you about earlier, it's possible to imbue your own meals with the same soul-satisfying connection to others.

In a similar spirit, when you're hosting a meal, ask one special guest to orchestrate the evening by creating a pleasurable atmosphere that ensures everyone present is honored and enjoys the occasion. An easy way for the evening's *magister bibendi* to accomplish this is to invite each guest to toast people, the food, or the event, perhaps every fifteen minutes or so, starting with the first course, then continuing through the main course and dessert. In this way, through the modern creative expression of an ancient tradition that embodies the best of friendship and shared spirits, you and your friends are creating your own time-honored ritual that encourages a welcoming and memorable meal for all. And now I would like to make another toast: to "friendship-flavored" food . . . all ways.

Create Multigenerational Meal-Memories

If there's one comment about her cooking that Anita Bellandi often made, it was, "No, it's not sauce, it's tomato *gravy*." Explains her granddaughter Vinita Azarow: "During a summertime job while in college, I lived with my Italian grandmother, *Nonna* Anita, in her flat in San Francisco's Marina district. When I arrived home for dinner, I would sometimes be greeted by the exquisitely familiar aroma of her tomato sauce. But, ask my grandmother if she was making tomato sauce (*salsa di pomodoro*), and in her Italian accent she would often respond, 'No, I'm making tomato *gravy*.'"

While most of us would describe Nonna's elixir as a sauce and not gravy, perhaps she had the original meaning of "gravy" in mind— for it initially signified a sort of spiced stock-based sauce; only in the sixteenth century did its meaning as a "sauce made from meat juices" emerge. More likely, the legacy of Nonna's tomato "gravy" has its roots in Italy, where various tomato-based recipes evolved to form the base of a soup, stew, or sauce. Sometimes ingredients consisted of *soffrito* (soh-FREE-toh), which literally means "under or barely fried," to describe finely minced carrots, celery, and onion that have been sautéed in olive oil. Optional additions include garlic, parsley, and a few leaves of fresh sage; if the recipe calls for it, pancetta (pan-CHEH-tuh), Italian bacon cured with salt, pepper, and other spices, but not smoked, may be included in a *soffritto*. Or another option could be *battuto* (bah-TOO-toh), *soffrito* without the olive oil sauté.

When I asked Vinita how she knew Nonna had made tomato gravy on certain days when she came home from her summer job, her response about the sensory ways in which it filled the flat was instant: "How do you describe that wonderful smell of the sauce cooking, the herbs, the basil, the garlic that went into it? There was a full flavor to it—not like prepared store-bought sauces that are overly tomato-y. Instead, Nonna's fresh ingredients and finely diced vegetables (some grown in her garden) created a rich underbase, a layering that was part of the complexity of the flavor."

Spicing the sauce with special social occasions also added to its flavor. "Nonna would make and serve her special sauce during those times when the family would come over to her home," reflects Vinita. "The table would glow with her best crystal, china, and hand-embroidered linen tablecloth." Clearly, her granddaughter's summer-long stay also warranted serving the special sauce. "We would sit in her dining nook and eat the sauce with other fresh food she would cook for us. The meal was served on dishes with pink roses, not far from the kitchen door that led to the garden. It's still a special memory," adds Vinita. (Chapter 7, "Unappetizing Atmosphere," offers insights into the benefits of an aesthetically set table.)[7]

As with the different generations of Italian-Americans in Roseto, Pennsylvania, eating and enjoying a meal together seemed to make a difference in the health and well-being of Nonna and her family. To create your own multigenerational memories:

- Start your own family tradition by inviting one or more family members over to enjoy a meal made with a recipe from an older member of your family—perhaps an aunt or uncle, parent, or cousin. As Nonna did during special holidays and occasions, set a glowing table with special ware.
- Create your own "family" by starting a cooking club. Invite coworkers, friends, and community members with whom you interact—such as a librarian, neighbors, and people you know who work in restaurants—to be part of your club. Rotate meals at the homes of different members. In the spirit of *tamada*, share meal-memories and stories as you dine.
- Make a favorite recipe, and then invite friends and family from different generations over for an informal meal.
- If you live alone, consider placing a picture of a family- or friendship-filled meal on the table as you eat; or, if there's a special meal your mother used to make that you especially enjoyed, make it for yourself on the weekend when you have some extra time, defrost it while you're at work, and then enjoy it when you get home, while, at the same time, you reflect on your family or friends as you eat.

Share Meaningful Meals . . . in Spirit

It's a fact: ancient Romans followed pagan customs by feasting and eating to excess. Only the worship of their more moderate, frugal ancestors, and of their many gods, served to curtail their gorging. Pagans believed that the gods depended on humans to create lodging for them in the form of temples and to feed them through food offerings. Thinking that extravagant temples and an abundance of food kept the gods in a good mood, the Romans were eager to acknowledge their presence by inviting them to join in the meal. Only after the gods were offered the first mouthfuls of food and the first drops of poured wine, did the Romans eat.

Nonna's Tomato Gravy

Recipe by Anita Giovacchini Bellandi and Vinita Bellandi Azarow

Prior to the latter half of the twentieth century, recipes that parents made for their families were often learned from *their* parents or other family members. Create your own culinary family tree and, therefore, a connection to your roots, both people- and food-wise, by putting together recipes from your own family. Here is Nonna's Tomato Gravy, which Vinita Azarow remembers fondly as a special after-school meal made specially for her by her grandmother. Says Vinita: "These amounts are approximate; my Nonna didn't measure her ingredients. As I watched her, I guessed at the amounts she was using. Add or take away according to your taste."

To put the meal together, make a simple meal of your favorite pasta, mixed together with Nonna's tomato gravy, which has been infused with the flavor of fresh, finely diced vegetables. Finally, don't forget to sprinkle it with freshly grated cheese. "Nonna was partial to Pecorino Romano, but Parmesan is also good," Vinata says. "She always served the pasta with fresh greens dressed with red wine vinegar and extra-virgin olive oil, with salt and pepper to taste. San Pellegrino water would be on the table. And dessert might consist of an apple, with a couple of her anisette cookies."

 1 to 2 tablespoons olive oil
 1 small onion, finely chopped
 $^1/_2$ stalk celery, finely chopped
 1 small carrot, finely chopped
 2 cloves garlic, finely chopped
 1 tablespoon finely chopped fresh parsley
 1 (28-ounce) can plum tomatoes

4 to 6 basil leaves, torn into smallish pieces
   (if using dried basil, use $^1/_2$ teaspoon and add it
   with the parsley)
Salt and pepper
Sugar
2 tablespoons butter

To make the *soffrito*, heat the olive oil over medium heat. Lower the heat, then sauté the onion for 5 to 7 minutes, or until lightly golden. Add the celery, carrot, garlic, and parsley and cook for 5 minutes, or until lightly browned. The garlic should turn a light golden color; be careful not to brown it. (Note: Nonna often deglazed the vegetables by adding some red wine and scraping up the browned bits before she added the plum tomatoes.)

Decrease the heat to low. Break apart the plum tomatoes with your hands, then add to the *soffrito*. Simmer for about 5 minutes. Add the basil and season with salt and pepper to taste. Add a bit of sugar to adjust the acidity of the tomatoes, if needed. Continue to simmer for about 20 minutes, or until the sauce has reached the desired thickness. When it's ready, the bubbles coming up will be a lighter orange color than the gravy.

Just before serving, stir in the butter.

Variation: Tomato gravy with meat. Vinita told me that sometimes Nonna would make the tomato gravy with meat. To do this, "she would brown a smashed clove of garlic first in the olive oil and then remove it. Then she would brown pieces of beef (which could be ground beef, ground veal, or pieces of steak) in the garlic-flavored olive oil. At that point she would remove the meat and deglaze the pan with a little wine (Marsala, or a good red that she would have on hand). After the pan was deglazed, she would proceed to cook the vegetables as above, adding the meat back in during the final simmer."

In the tradition of the ancient Romans, even though many of us eat alone, it is still possible to share food with friends and family members . . . in spirit. To make your own meaningful connection, just prior to eating, think of a family member, friend, or person you admire (living or not). Then, while thinking of this person—and perhaps also of a meaningful memory you shared—place a small portion of food from your plate on a separate, small plate positioned next to your table setting. In the spirit of honoring ancestors, also add a drop or two of your beverage of choice to the plate. Just before eating, close your eyes and inhale and exhale slowly as you reminiscence about your friend or family member. Throughout the meal, eat *from* your heart (see chapter 8, "Sensory Disregard," for more about this) by continuing to reflect on the much-valued person.

Family Fare for the Twenty-First Century

My friend Mary called one day to tell me about a new concept of family meals she had just read about in our local newspaper. Knowing how time-pressured so many heads-of-household are, some women had gotten together to provide "everything you need to assemble delicious dinners for your family, store in the freezer and then serve in the weeks ahead." To reap the convenience, all homemakers have to do is call or just stop by the store to order their meals and then pick up the fresh ingredients, already prepped, at their convenience. All they have to do when they get home is assemble the ingredients and then cook them. *Voilà!* Dinner is served.[8]

If such a service is a dream you don't think you can afford, or if it simply isn't available in your area, consider doing the same service for yourself by asking for assistance from family members or friends. Pick a day, set aside some time, and then plan your meals for the week. Shop for your ingredients, and then either assemble and prep them all in advance, or, if you prefer, assemble and cook each meal independently, as the need arises.

Eat the Enlightened Diet Way

Chapter 10, "In Action," is filled with practical guidelines for putting all seven elements of the Enlightened Diet into action each day. As you practice the antidotes (see the section "Elemental Overview"), each of the weight-loss solutions that nourish body, mind, soul, and social well-being discussed throughout this book, you'll automatically and instinctively connect to food, others, and yourself. As you do, you'll be enriching your meals so that making food and eating doesn't *feel* like solo dining. To begin, create connection to both the food and yourself by making each meal an eating meditation (see chapter 3, "Task Snacking," for more about mindfulness meditation). To nourish yourself with the Enlightened Diet, focus on your food choices, preparing the meal, eating it, and then cleaning up afterward.

Overcoming Solo Dining

The antidote to the solo dining eating style is taking a cue from Europeans, ancient Romans, and state-of-the-art science, and deciding to dine and to share food experiences with others—either literally or in memory—as often as possible; to share a fresh meal or snack with colleagues, coworkers, family, or friends. As simple as the eating style of solo dining may seem, it is a two-edged sword in that it can be both easy and difficult to implement—especially with the demands of home, family, and career, and contending with cellular phones, pagers, and ongoing e-mail that keep us on call seemingly twenty-four hours a day. But the rewards are well worth the effort. The next chapter, "Unappetizing Atmosphere," also brings people into the eating experience, but in another way: through the psychological and aesthetic environment they create when you eat. The key concept is to turn a dining milieu that may not be pleasant into one that is warm, welcoming . . . and weight friendly.

Chapter 7

Unappetizing
Atmosphere

R̶x : Dine in psychologically and aesthetically
pleasing surroundings.

Both the *psychological* and the *aesthetic* atmospheres in which you dine hold the power to influence your weight and well-being. What do we mean by psychological and aesthetic atmospheres? Have you ever eaten in an especially pleasant place, surrounded by supportive people, convivial conversation, and classy accoutrements? Perhaps it was a special occasion, and your friends took you to a welcoming restaurant for your birthday; because they had organized the meal to celebrate you, the evening crackled with joy, conversation, and laughter.

The *external* mood, tone, and ambiance that surrounds you while eating determines the psychological atmosphere. In the example of the birthday party, it is celebratory and a source of pleasure. The milieu has an agreeable effect on you psychologically, as you and your friends chat convivially over a delicious meal; in response, your heart is open, and your soul is singing.

But the psychological atmosphere can also be negative, stress-filled, and unpleasant. Have you ever eaten while being scolded or criticized? Or in your car while driving during rush hour? Or while watching a horror movie or murder mystery on TV? If so, then you have had the experience of eating in an unpleasant psychological atmosphere. The surroundings in which you ate were so hectic or unpleasant that it affected your mind or mental processes in some way—either consciously (which would happen when you're being scolded while eating, for example) or unconsciously (you might not be aware of the impact that a horror movie, for instance, is having on your psyche or digestive process).

The other key component of the unpleasant atmosphere eating style is the aesthetics that surround you when you eat. Simply put, is the place in which you're dining welcoming in appearance—or not? If you're sitting on a hard plastic bench, if you're eating on a garishly colored plastic tabletop, with damp paper plates and plastic utensils, surely your dining aesthetics are unpleasant. Or perhaps you're eating on the run in a noisy fast food restaurant, with rock music blaring and fluorescent lighting glaring overhead. These are examples of aesthetically unpleasant surroundings.

As a contrast, envision a place with an agreeable atmosphere; for instance, as you arrive at a friend's home for a meal, you're greeted by the aroma of freshly prepared food cooking in the kitchen; you take a break from work at your favorite local café to enjoy the brew that the barista makes for you, personally; or during a special celebratory occasion, you enter an upscale restaurant that glows with glistening crystal chandeliers, a crisp, white tablecloth, and the murmur of quiet conversation; or maybe the soft candlelight makes you aware that the wooden dining table has a lovely patina that peeks out from pleasing placemats that are set with cloth napkins and quality utensils.

Whether appealing or appalling, both the psychological mood and the physical accessories that surround you when you eat may influence the way in which you metabolize food and, in turn, your health and well-being. Both the psychological and the aesthetic atmospheres that surround you when you eat are *externally* based, and both somehow impact your psyche and the way in which you metabolize meals.

You may find it amazing to consider that the atmosphere in which you eat may make a difference in your weight, but it does. This eating style is powerful in that, once you implement its antidotes, it may quickly improve the quality of your life by enhancing how you feel—both physically and emotionally; as another side effect, it may even improve your relationships—with others as well as with food. With this eating style, you will focus on the psychological and physical aesthetics of your food life; the atmosphere in your home, in restaurants, and at drive-thru restaurants; and the *quality* of companionship when you dine with family, friends, and coworkers—or by yourself. By this I mean, when you eat alone, are you taking the time to set a sumptuous table, play enjoyable music, and eat with a meditative mindset? Or are you eating pizza directly out of the cardboard box in which it was delivered, with the TV blasting in the background, distracted by the details of daily life? In other words, are *you* providing nice company for yourself?

Enchanting Ingredients

Long before our research revealed the psychological and aesthetic ingredients of the unpleasant atmosphere eating style as a risk factor for weight gain, we had clues that the atmosphere in which we eat somehow makes a difference to our psyche and, in turn, our health and well-being. One of the more memorable and exceptional dining environments we've experienced, one that brought a glow to both heart and soul (and palate), awaited us in our private dining room at Statholdergaarden in Oslo, Norway, the restaurant of award-winning chef Bent Stiansen. When Larry, our Norwegian friends Erik and Tine, and I entered the foyer, we were greeted by an elegant, Continental atmosphere, replete with chandeliers, the faint glow of candlelit tables, Oriental rugs covering polished wooden floors, portrait and landscape oil paintings on the walls, and the quiet conversation of elegantly garbed diners seated at antique wooden tables in the restaurant's various cozy dining rooms.

Just as delightful was the six-course vegetarian menu that lay like a crisp fall leaf at each place setting, and the solicitous, gracious waiters who presented the meal to us. Such a start was a prelude of things to come. Over the next five hours (yes, the meal lasted for five hours), course after course was served caringly and attentively. Surely, this was more than a meal, we realized; it was an extraordinary dining event. Throughout the enchanted evening, waiters glided in and out, unobtrusively. The only time they joined our conversation was at the beginning of each course, which they took the time to tell us about.

It's been more than five years since our memorable meal in Norway. Since then, we've eaten at many exceptional restaurants; even so, that evening at Statholdergaarden, surrounded by exceptional service, food, and friendship, still stands out as fare for heart and soul. And without a doubt, the enchanting psychological and aesthetic environs had a lot to do with the total nourishment of the evening, which, we have no doubt, will last a lifetime.

While our culinary experience in Norway was quite exceptional, we have experienced comparable Enlightened Diet dining experiences during everyday meals with friends at their homes, in local hole-in-the-wall restaurants we found serendipitously that served sublime food, and in meals we have made in our own home. For instance, the homemade meals prepared by our friends David Leivick and Linda Gibbs, in their seaside home in Northern California, always sparkle with freshness, flavor, David's creativity, and his love of cooking; the food we ate at a Thai restaurant we stumbled on before going to a local movie on a rainy Sunday afternoon was so delicious and authentic we felt we were in Thailand; and the potluck Thanksgiving meals in our home that are the culmination of friends' specialties (Peter's ten-ingredient salads are meals in themselves; Penny's cranberry sauce is a holiday luxury; and Vinita makes really mean desserts) have also been memorable.

In contrast to our psychologically and aesthetically satisfying, exceptional, epicurean Norwegian meal, Americans currently eat about

20 percent of their meals inside their cars—often between errands or meetings. To accommodate this growing group, the fast food outlet In-N-Out Burger has developed paper "laptops" so that we can keep our clothes clean while we drive and eat. Whether surrounded by car fumes, fluorescent lights, or loud, abrasive noise, dining frequently in an unpleasant atmosphere contributes to a negative relationship with food and increased odds of growing girth. What the dining experience we had in Norway tells us is that food technology and what, how, and where we eat may have changed over the years, but the type of surroundings that hold the power to nourish our soul when we dine has not. What happens when the opposite is the norm, when the atmosphere in which we eat is typically jarring to the psyche? When both the psychological and the aesthetic surroundings are not only unwelcoming and unpleasant, but they're also overtly hostile? An unusual study that was done just after World War II can give us some clues.

Hostile Ingredients

On June 16, 1951, the prestigious medical journal *The Lancet* published a study that could not be done today. Not only were children involved, but the conditions were also so health-threatening—both emotionally and physically—that a modern-day review board would never approve the study design. The year was 1948 when British nutritionist Elsie M. Widdowson worked at orphanages in Germany, where thousands of children were orphaned casualties of World War II. Having lost their families, it was a time of extreme trauma for the orphans; needless to say, their suffering and deprivation was exacerbated by food shortages and rationing.

While working at two orphanages, Widdowson had the wherewithal to observe and record an extraordinary situation that evolved. Her one-year study started when she decided to monitor and measure the impact of additional servings of food on the children's weight and height. Would those who received food in addition to their rations gain more weight than those who received rations only? Would they grow and gain more height than children who ate lesser amounts of food? To find out, during the first six months of the study, Widdowson gave children at both orphanages equal food portions; during the second six-month period, she fed children at one orphanage larger portions of bread, jam, and orange juice. Throughout the twelve months of the study, she weighed and measured the height of the children every ten days.

When the time came to look at the height and weight charts, Widdowson was perplexed at what she found: during the first six months, when children at both orphanages received equal food portions, children at one orphanage had gained a lot more weight, and had grown much more, than children at the other orphanage. The results became even more confounding when she realized that the children at the orphanage who had been fed more food during the second six-month period gained *less* weight and height than those who had been fed lesser amounts of food. To solve the mystery, Widdowson pondered at first whether it was possible for children to thrive—or not—regardless of the quantity of food they ate. But when she scrutinized the atmosphere in both orphanages, she got an unexpected explanation for the seemingly contradictory results: Frau Schwarz, the children's caretaker. Each group of children who had failed to gain weight and grow had been overseen by a strict disciplinarian who chose mealtime to publicly ridicule and rebuke certain children; this explained the difference. "By the time she had finished," writes Widdowson, "all the children would be in a state of considerable agitation, and several of them might be in tears."

Have you ever felt hungry, then lost your appetite because you were upset? Or did food ever sit like a lump because you ate while agitated? Or perhaps you've eaten to stuff down feelings. The idea that your psychological state can influence digestion is now so familiar that it is easy to lose sight of how amazing Widdowson's findings were. But amazing they are. After all, the discovery that children's psychological surroundings when they eat can impact their metabolism to such a degree that it determines whether they gain weight and grow is remarkable. It also leads us to the question, does a stress-filled environment influence the way we digest and metabolize food and, in turn, influence our health and well-being? Answering this question calls for a rudimentary understanding of the process of digestion and the role that atmosphere and, in turn, emotions, can play.[1]

The Link Between Stress and Poor Digestion

One of the most remarkable stories of how emotions can affect digestion starts in 1822, on Mackinac Island in Michigan, when an army surgeon named William Beaumont, who was stationed at Fort Mackinac, treated eighteen-year-old French Canadian fur trapper Alexis St. Martin for an accidental gunshot wound to his stomach. Shot at close range, St. Martin's injury was so serious that Beaumont didn't expect him to survive. But he did. And then, in a unique turn of events, not only did St. Martin live, but the major wound also healed, except for a small opening in his stomach that never closed.

At the time, little was known about the process of digestion; it was a mystery that was discussed and debated in the medical community in Europe, especially in France. Ignorant of the debate that raged, but intrigued by the puzzle of digestion, Beaumont turned St. Martin's mishap into groundbreaking observational studies: over a period of ten years, during which time he performed about two hundred experiments, he became the first medical scientist to observe and carefully record the digestive process of a human being. What exactly occurred when food was digested? What were the elements of stomach acid? Beaumont documented it all. From these observations, he was the first to show that digestion actually slowed down when St. Martin was upset. How did this remarkable first-time observation come about? Because Beaumont's observational studies were time consuming and difficult and, well, unpleasant and difficult to endure, St. Martin would become irritated. For instance, the only way Beaumont could observe digestion was to place food via a silk string into the opening in St. Martin's stomach and then remove it to observe any changes. And it was during one of these experiments that Beaumont observed that the food was not digested as well when St. Martin was upset.[2]

Since Beaumont's pioneering observations, science has made great strides in decoding the emotions-digestion puzzle—what behavioral scientists, today, might describe as the mind-body connection. Consider what happens when you eat while stressed, which was what happened to the children in Widdowson's experiment who failed to grow or gain weight. Before I tell you more about the impact that a stressful psychological environment can have on your digestion and weight, it will be helpful for you to know that there are many definitions of "stress"; I'm defining it as a "perceived threat" to either physical or emotional well-being.

Why does it matter whether you eat while stressed out, when you're experiencing unpleasant emotions? When you do, your brain releases a torrent of sometimes contradictory hormones (naturally occurring chemical messengers) that put your digestive system in disarray. For instance, to give you strength for "fight or flight" in response to a perceived threat, you may manufacture the fat-friendly hormone *cortisol*, or CRH (*corticotrophin*-releasing hormone), which in turn produces energy-giving adrenaline (which will give you the energy to sprint or struggle). CRH has other potentially powerful effects. It can also suppress your appetite (which is what seems to have happened to Widdowson's upset orphans), or it may have the opposite impact: it may produce steroids (an organic fat-soluble compound) that can make you *hungry*. If this happens, your mind-body may prompt you to satisfy your hunger by overeating calorie-dense foods such as cookies, cake, or potato chips. In other words, an unpleasant psychological atmosphere when you're eating can cause your body to produce hormones that prompt you to eat more; ergo, the mind-body link to weight gain.

Mealtime Emotions

Why have we been created with an amazingly strong connection between the brain and the digestive system, with a relationship between our surroundings and digestion that is so powerful and integral to our well-being and survival that the stomach and intestines are abundant in nerve cells—with even more than the spinal cord? Why has our mind-body been designed to pay such close attention to our environment and our emotions, with the ability to respond accordingly, including when we're eating? Research by Candace B. Pert, which explores the physical, emotional, and spiritual reasons for feelings, can give us some clues.

Pert's pioneering work is especially relevant to a discussion about the impact of eating in a psychologically and aesthetically unpleasant atmosphere because it presents a scientific picture about how environment may influence digestion and increase your drive to overeat; in other words: stress more, eat more. The story starts with substances called *peptides*, which reside not only in the brain but also throughout your entire body. And it is *neuropeptides*, specifically, that act as the biological foundation of the awareness we bring to meals; indeed, to all aspects of our lives.

What is especially unique about neuropeptides is that they are released into the bloodstream by *nerve cells*. The link to nerve cells is especially fascinating because the hormones and other chemicals that our mind-body makes create a two-way freeway that serves as a dynamic information network between the brain and the digestive system. In other words, neuropeptides influence your experience of your world; and vice versa, your consciousness, or mind, or emotions, affect your biology, or body. Put another way, your body is strongly influenced by your emotions. Because of this, "the environment in which you eat has a lot to do with your emotional experience at mealtime," writes Pert. Eat in an unappetizing atmosphere, and "it's a kind of disintegration, *a mind-body split that will lead to weight gain* [italics mine] and disease conditions caused . . . by incomplete digestion."[3]

But there's another reason you're likely to eat more and gain weight when you consume food in an unpleasant psychological atmosphere: it influences the type (worse) and quantity (more) of food you eat. Researchers discovered this relationship when they asked thirty subjects to watch *Love Story*, a sad movie that leads people to cry easily and often. As the study subjects watched the movie, they ate 28 percent more (124.97 grams versus 97.97 grams) buttered, salty popcorn than they did while watching *Sweet Home Alabama*, a breezy comedy.[4] The same researchers found similar results with college students who were asked to read about little children who died in a fire. As they read the sad, disturbing, and heartbreaking news, they ate four times more M&M's than raisins from nearby bowls of snacks. In contrast, when the same students read about a delightful chance reunion among four old friends, they *didn't* turn to unhealthful food, but rather to good-tasting snacks. The key message: refrain from using the dinner table as a place to argue or to scold or to think about unpleasant people or situations if you want to eat less and weigh less.

Food and Fuel

Earlier in this chapter, I told you about orphaned children who were subjected to an abusive atmosphere while they ate. But there are plenty of situations that lend themselves to an aesthetically unpleasant and discordant eating atmosphere. Consider this common scenario: You're driving in your car in Anywhere, USA. Realizing you need to buy gas, you pull into a nearby gas station, next to a gas tank. When you get out of your car to fuel up, a sign tells you that you need to pay inside first. As you walk past other motorists who are filling their tanks, you visibly cringe, albeit slightly, as you register the unpleasant, potent smell of petroleum that surrounds you. Feeling a bit queasy from the odor, when you walk inside the store to prepay, your nostrils are instantly filled with the scent of rancid cooking oil; at the same time, the harshness of the overhead fluorescent light causes you to squint a bit. While waiting in line to pay the cashier, you glance at the small TV on the counter near the cashier that is blasting bad news. You're also privy to a distasteful discussion between the cashier and the customer in front of you, who claims he has been short-changed. To fill the time, you look around to locate the source of the unappetizing aroma that greeted you. Instantly, you realize it's coming from a fast food outlet that is sharing space within the gasoline station's store. At the same time, you notice that a customer who just walked out the door toward his car is eating a hamburger and fries he bought from the outlet. He'll probably eat it while driving, you think, while continuing to wait.

Such "cobranded on-site locations"—the merger of a fast food outlet and a gas station, or two or more fast food restaurants under one roof—is a common sight and eating experience for many Americans. Think, for a moment, about the last gas station store you entered that was abundant with packaged junk food, the last fast food restaurant where you ate, or the last open-all-night convenience store you went to for a late-night snack. In how many of those cases were you aware of the unappetizing atmosphere, the subtle assault it was making on your psyche, and the way in which it was impacting your digestive system, indeed, your entire being?

Optimal Healing Environments

Although it's an emerging field, more and more the medical community is becoming aware that environment has a profound impact on health and healing. The movement is gaining such momentum that, at the second Symposium on Optimal Healing Environments sponsored by the Samueli Institute, physician and author Larry Dossey described the study of healing environments as a "'huge social movement' whose momentum is unstoppable." Indeed, a newsletter on the topic said that more than fifty scientists and clinicians were invited to the event to define "healing environments" and challenges related to creating them.

Intrigued, I studied the symposium's topics, which addressed environments for disciplines as diverse as nursing, Integrative Medicine, and health care in general, as well as for ailments ranging from chronic cardiovascular disease and chronic low-back pain to cancer and childhood obesity. Given our own research and the unappetizing atmosphere eating style we identified, the presentation that really caught my attention was the work of Marc Schweitzer and colleagues because it identified specific elements in the environment that make an impact on health. "The 'ambiance' of a space has an effect on people using the space," Schweitzer states. And then he goes on to identify elements that are integral to a healing environment: personal space; sound/noise; temperature; fresh air and ventilation; enjoyable social interaction (social support); warm, natural light; color; a view and experience of nature; arts, esthetics, and entertainment (such as music).[5]

I was especially interested in Schweitzer's overview of the elements of a healing environment that have so far been identified, because throughout this chapter I'm suggesting that the atmosphere in which you eat can be healing—by increasing the odds of optimal digestion and, in turn, optimal weight and well-being—or harmful—by increasing the odds of poor digestion or overeating, thus contributing to weight gain. After all, as we have seen, throughout the day you have plenty of nonhealing opportunities to assault your psyche and system (and waistline) by eating in an abrasive atmosphere, such as in the gas station store situation I described above. If you recall, it was replete with harsh lighting, contrary people, and depressing news blaring from the TV. Add cramped quarters, stuffy and stale air, and a motley collection of disparate, disconnected, and cluttered food products and car accoutrements, and you have the antithesis of the healing environment that Schweitzer's research revealed.

Optimal Eating Atmosphere

Most of us know that eating in congenial surroundings is, at the very least, enjoyable. This is especially good news, since you can access or create delightful surroundings any time. For instance, envision a fall picnic, surrounded by the bittersweet mood of autumn, as the colors of the season materialize both in the leaves on trees and in the deep orange of pumpkin soup. Or think of the soothing serenity and comfort of a homemade stew that you eat in winter as candlelight flickers on the dining table and you're surrounded by steamed-up windows, while outside, a blanket of snow covers your yard. Or imagine an impromptu meal of improvised pasta, sauce, salad, and wine that you make with friends, when a sudden spring shower abates. Or picture a summer salad that you sprinkle with edible and organic flowers, such as squash blossoms. The possibilities are endless. Yet the role that ambiance and your surroundings play in overeating and weight gain (as well as indigestion problems) continues to be an overlooked aspect of optimal eating and well-being.

In addition to the many ideas I've discussed in this chapter (such as the enchanting ingredients inherent in the dining experience we had at Statholdergaarden in Norway), I have created a rich repository of other strategies for accessing the nourishing aspect of dining in a relaxing, delightful, aesthetically likable, and welcoming atmosphere—ideas you can use to reenact.

What would an optimal psychological and aesthetic eating environment look like? Here are some suggestions for creating an affable dining milieu . . . as often as possible.

Limit lighting. One of our favorite restaurants has low hanging lights above each booth, which we find to be harsh. Each time we eat there, we think about how much more we would enjoy the meal and the entire dining experience if, instead, it were infused with candlelight. When you eat at home, diffuse the light by turning on a favorite nearby lamp, dimming your overhead light, or eating by candlelight.

Walk away. A friend of mine told me that not too long after she read our research paper on the eating styles, she was feeling hypoglycemic (weak from low blood sugar) and hungry in the middle of the day while "choring." So she made the spontaneous decision to buy a sweet from a gourmet cookie shop to quickly appease her hunger. But the acid rock music that blasted from speakers, and the uninterested clerks who continued to talk among themselves instead of taking her order, dissuaded her from staying. She found a friendlier place down the block for a midday munch. When you eat out—whether it's a full meal or a munchie—choose an amiable place whenever possible.

Cherish china. When Oprah did a show on "anti-aging breakthroughs," a weight loss lifestyle was one of the topics. To highlight the elements of her successful weight loss, an audience member shared her personal success story. Along with moving more and choosing fresh food, the aesthetic atmosphere she created was part of her successful twenty-two-pound weight loss. "I put my portion [of food] on beautiful plates, with great style, lovely linens, crystal, [and] china, and enjoyed every morsel," she said. "No more standing in the kitchen eating out of a little container."[6] Whenever possible, eat on quality plates, with the best utensils you have, and sit down at a dining table to enjoy your meal even more.

Rest, relax. A friend of ours who is a *yogini* (a woman who practices yoga), told us that after she shared a large lunch in the home of a revered family in India, her hosts invited her to lie down and rest so that she could digest the meal in a peaceful and quiet environment. In a time- and work-driven country like ours, this isn't a realistic option, but what we *can* do is a modified version: after eating, take the time to enjoy some easygoing, postprandial conversation with others, some relaxing music, or an enjoyable article.

Release emotions. Because of Candace Pert's research on emotions and digestion, it is safe to say that the psychological atmosphere in which you eat influences the way you metabolize food and, in turn, your weight and well-being. That's why you'll find it helpful to release toxic molecules of emotion when you eat. To do this, if you find that you're ruminating about something unpleasant, put your emotions on hold and press the pause button as you eat; instead, think about something agreeable. You can always return to the problem later. Or, if the people with whom you're dining are more negative than positive, try to redirect the conversation by asking them to share something that is working well or is enjoyable in their lives.

Eat outside. If there's a park near your house, some outdoor dining tables and chairs in the courtyard where you work, or a café that enables you to eat while outdoors as you enjoy some fresh air and beautiful surroundings, take advantage of the opportunity. And there's another benefit: you can get some exercise while walking to your favorite outdoor eating place. (See chapter 9, "Enlightened Exercise," for ideas about including more motion and movement in your life.)

Overcoming Unappetizing Atmosphere

I wasn't surprised when our research revealed unappetizing atmosphere as an eating style linked with overeating. What astonished me was that, as with all the eating styles, it was statistically significant; in other words, it's not due to chance. The psychological and aesthetic environments connected to food and eating may be the most overlooked aspect of weight gain, but, as we've seen throughout this chapter, it is a powerful determinant of your weight. To increase your odds of achieving and maintaining optimal weight, we've given you lots of guidelines for dining in psychologically and aesthetically pleasing surroundings that are inherently healing and healthy. In the next chapter, "Sensory Disregard," we reveal yet another "invisible" eating style: the price your mind-body and waistline pay when you disregard the sensory and spiritual nutrients in food. You will also discover insights into the benefits of these spiritual ingredients, and how you can turn each food experience into a soul-satisfying success.

Chapter 8

Sensory Disregard

℞ : Savor flavors when you eat.

We had the opportunity to experience the power of savoring flavors while eating long before we identified sensory disregard as one of the eating styles. It was while we were having dinner in a beautiful Thai restaurant, where we had ordered a salad with which we were not familiar. Called *miang kam*, the dish that arrived at our table wasn't the familiar American salad of mixed vegetables; instead, we were presented with a platter that held six small bowls, each filled with finely chopped and colorful ingredients: lime, peanuts, red onion, red pepper, ginger, and roasted coconut. In the center were a bunch of fresh spinach leaves and another bowl of a very thick and sticky sweet-and-sour paste. The presentation was enchanting, but because it was also unfamiliar, we asked our waitress how to proceed. Patiently, she showed us how to take one spinach leaf, spread a little paste on it, and sprinkle a tiny portion from each bowl over the paste. Then she created a small food-filled tube by rolling up the spinach leaf. When we tasted the handmade tubular salad, like a fireworks display, our taste buds burst with flavor. With each bite, an implosion of flavors was released, so much so that we kept our attention and our anticipation focused on the fantastic flavors and tantalizing tastes that each new *miang kam* released.

Sensory Disregard–Spiritual Disconnection

Our dining experience with *miang kam* is an exceptional example of how fresh food that has been prepared with care and savored by the diners can fill the senses and satisfy the soul—the two key ingredients lacking in the sensory disregard eating style. We are especially excited to tell you about this eating style because our research is the first to reveal the sensory and spiritual elements—which go together like twins—of eating . . . and of overeating. When you take time to experience your food through all your senses—taste (flavor), smell (aroma), sight (presentation), sound (of surroundings), and touch (kinesthetics)—and to regard the mystery of life inherent in both food and yourself, you're more likely to be truly nourished, and less likely to overeat. In other words, dining with your senses (sensory *regard*) while at the same time eating with a deep appreciation for the food before you (spiritual *connection*) are powerful ways to nurture and nourish yourself and, in turn, to feel fulfilled by the dining experience. When you take the time to do this, you're more likely to eat less and enjoy it more.

Such regard and connection to eating is the antithesis of how many who struggle with weight relate to food. What is more typical is sensory *dis*regard and spiritual *dis*connection. What does this eating style look like? If you've ever eaten quickly and mindlessly (more about this in chapter 4, "Emotional Eating") and scarfed down food because, perhaps, you've let yourself become superhungry or, say, you're feeling depressed and your emotions are dictating what and how you're eating, then you've eaten without experiencing the color of the food, its aroma, flavors, texture, presentation, and portion size; this is sensory disregard. At the same time, if you typically eat without reflecting on the mystery of food's ability to sustain life; if you ignore the way in which the elements, such as rain, sunshine, wind, and soil, work together to create the fruits, vegetables, whole grains, legumes, and nuts and seeds, as well as dairy, eggs, fish, poultry, and meat, that nourish you; and if you eat without savoring and appreciating, from the heart, the origins of the food before you—then you are eating with spiritual disconnection.

The idea that eating with sensory disregard and spiritual disconnection can lead to weight gain, it must be said, may seem somewhat unusual. After all, the straightforward and seemingly simple one-size-fits-all, calories in–calories out formula discussed in chapter 2, "Food Fretting," is the standard solution to weight loss that most health professionals stand by: just cut down on the amount of food you eat, and move more, and you'll lose weight. Eating with your senses and connecting to the meaning in meals, on the other hand, isn't so straightforward and simple. Rather, it requires you to replace calorie counting with sensory and sensual pleasure, and to transform phobic food thoughts ("I can't eat that; it's fattening") into a world filled with the wonder and delight of food and eating, and into a relationship with food that includes appreciating the meaning and mystery of life inherent in your meals.

Surely most of us *don't* flavor our meals with sensory and spiritual delight. And we're paying a big price for it with our growing girth. While vacationing in Mexico, Mark Morford, a columnist at the *San Francisco Chronicle*, observed many overweight Americans; he considered the sensory and spiritual starvation that is normal for many Americans, and its link with being overweight. Such thoughts prompted him to speculate about the detachment so many overweight people must feel from their bodies, a spiritual emptiness and lack of true nourishment—even as they're overeating.[1]

You can fill a sense of spiritual vacuity, a lack of true nourishment each time you eat, if you take the time to taste your food and to appreciate the multidimensional ways it nourishes you; in other words, if you take the time to savor the flavors in your food.

Sacred Scents

A time-tested example of the way in which humankind has for millennia turned to the senses to satisfy the soul is Judaism's sacred scents ceremony. Toward dusk, after a Saturday of resting, thinking, reading, or playing (just *being* rather than *doing*), the Jewish Sabbath ends when three stars can be seen in the sky. This transition—between the Sabbath and the other days of the week—is also celebrated with blessings. Called havdalah, meaning "separation," the informal farewell calls for a wine cup filled with wine, a candle, and a box filled with spices (*besamin*).

"May the coming week overflow with goodness like the wine in the cup," says the head of the household, holding the *kiddish* cup as it brims with wine. Then a special candle, made of twisted strands that symbolize the many different kinds of light God created (the light of the sun, moon, and stars, and the Jewish laws by which to live), is lit. Next, a spice box (a replacement for the incense-burning of ancient times) is opened, releasing the fragrant scent of cloves, nutmeg, and bay leaves. The symbolism: hope for a week that will be pleasant and sweet smelling.

Judaism's havdalah ceremony, which signifies the end of Shabbat, is a brief service that is rich in the inhalation of sweet and savory spices. Its purpose is to capture the senses and serve as a reminder to hold on to moments of sweetness and peace during the busy work week. Such symbolism has its roots in the *neshama yeterah*, the second, extra soul Jews are believed to acquire during Shabbat, which enhances the ability to rejoice in tranquility, and to live filled with a feeling of contentment. Indeed, the holiness and intention of the day is one of *oneg Shabbat*—the joy, pleasure, relaxation, and ease of the Sabbath.

When Shabbat draws to a close, tradition holds that the extra soul withdraws, leaving the mundane soul in its place. Because it's believed that aromas from the material world are the only aspect that the everyday, remaining soul can enjoy, the spice box and its scents serve to console and connect with the remaining soul throughout the week. In this way, inhaling the sacred aromatics signifies more than the moment of transition from the spiritual to the material world as the Sabbath ends: it also fills our being with the spicy sweetness of each moment. And, as these sacred scents capture the senses and provide a mindful pause, we are empowered to hold on to the peaceful, meaningful memory of the Sabbath—until next Friday at sunset.

Flavor Full Weight Loss

Perhaps Judaism's havdalah ceremony evolved with the intuitive understanding that slowing down and taking the time to savor scents is one path to spiritual satisfaction. But might it lead to weight loss, as our study on the seven eating styles suggests? Perhaps the best example of the way in which "eating with your senses" may successfully lead to weight loss is evident in the work of psychologist Seth Roberts, a professor of psychology at the University of California, Berkeley. While reviewing scientific journals in preparation for a lecture, Roberts had an "aha!" insight: Is it possible, he wondered, that the amount of body fat you have is linked to—even controlled by—the flavor in the food you eat? Somehow, might the brain depend on the flavor in food to gauge how much fat your body stores (leading to weight gain) or releases (leading to weight loss)?[2]

At the time, Roberts's reasoning was derived from insights into human beings' ancient evolution as well as state-of-the-art brain research.[3] Isn't it likely, he thought, that when we eat a lot of tasty, tempting, high-calorie food (such as ice cream, donuts, or potato chips), our brain thinks this is a time of abundance (translation: a caveman has just killed a tiger, and food will be plentiful for a while); then, to ensure you'll survive during times of scarcity, your brain tells your body to stockpile the pounds you put on from the food and to hold on to them. In essence, Roberts is saying that flavorful food triggers "an increase in hunger and fat storage. By contrast, not-so-mouthwatering or flavorless calories signal scarcity." He is suggesting that when you consume simple, unflavored food (he uses cooking oil, such as canola, as an example, but iceberg lettuce, steamed rice, or air-popped popcorn also illustrate the idea), your brain gets the message that you're not too hungry and therefore you eat less, making it easy for stored fat to be released.[4]

To put his interesting idea into action, Roberts used his own mind-body . . . and taste buds. In fact, my friend and colleague, Keri Brenner, who is a journalist and author with a specialty in health and Complementary and Alternative Medicine (CAM), interviewed Roberts for an article she wrote about his Shangri-La Diet. Brenner was interested in writing about Roberts's work because he claimed he had lost fifty pounds by having either a tablespoon of oil between meals or a cup of water sweetened with one tablespoon of sugar (fructose). He also told Brenner he actually had to gain back ten pounds, because over a long period of time he had become too thin. Now, to maintain his weight loss, he eats one meal a day, with small snacks such as fruit during the day, still taking the oil or sugar-water, but not as frequently—and he claims he isn't hungry for any more than that.

Does Roberts's flavor-based theory hold up? Intrigued by a newspaper article she read about Roberts's plan, Brenner decided to find out. "I thought it was unusual and interesting, because it's not a traditional diet," she told me, "and it doesn't involve any special menus or calorie counting; there's no exercise, or any of the other usual weight loss 'suspects.'" She was also interested in the Shangri-La Diet for personal reasons. "I've always struggled with the usual extra five or ten pounds," she said, citing a common problem for women. Brenner has dabbled with different diets and exercise regimens over the years to lose the extra weight. Could the "no hunger, eat anything, weight loss plan" espoused by Roberts really make a difference? Here's Brenner's experience:

I gave up baked goods and bread seven years ago, because
I have a predisposition to overeat refined carbs and sugars
and then gain weight. And I don't feel good. Roberts's plan was
appealing because it sounded simple and easy. All I had to do
to follow his program was to take measured doses of dull,
unflavored food, such as one cup of fructose-flavored water,
or one tablespoon of flavorless extra-light olive oil, in between
meals, two to four times a day; you can do either one. As part
of the plan, I also couldn't eat or drink or even brush my teeth
with peppermint toothpaste, an hour before or after taking the
oil or sugar-water, so that I wouldn't contaminate my palate with
other tastes.

During the first week after I started the diet, I was in a
restaurant with my husband, and the grilled fish and salad
combination arrived. I took a bite, and I knew I was actually
meditating. It was that intense. My whole mouth was filled with
the flavor of the food, and the experience of eating was much
richer, more intense, and satisfying than usual. I was almost
experiencing the chef preparing the food, all the care that went
into creating these flavors; I had an appreciation of the food in
every way. I remember thinking that somebody really put a lot of
regard and care into the food. When I took a bite, I was instantly
connected to the whole creation of the food; much more so than
normal. And I think I experienced this because it was such a
strong contrast to the flavorless food. It was transcendent; truly.

Did the plan take away my hunger? Absolutely, it did—
[especially] for mindless snacking. But I would be hungry for
healthy food—salads, proteins, and other fresh foods. Then,
when I would eat a meal, I had a much greater appreciation for
the flavors in the food. When I ate, I seemed to experience more
pleasure and awareness. I would take a bite, and the flavor
would be intensified. As a consequence, I ate less because I felt
more satisfied when I ate, because I appreciated the flavors in
the food. I also ate more fresh food. For me, Roberts's theory

works. I lost four or five pounds during the first month, without trying. I also lost my appetite for random snacking and grazing on nuts, trail mix, and protein bars while at work. On the other hand, I gained a greater appreciation of fresh food, and how it tasted. I stopped eating on autopilot and started to look forward to deliberately paying attention to what I was eating, and to the flavors. I wasn't trying to do this; it just happened.

Brenner told me she followed the plan for about three months but tapered off after a while, because her schedule got too hectic. She just didn't have the time to continue taking the oil and sugar-water supplements. Soon, she got out of the habit of supplementing with oil or sugar water during the day. And when she returned to her regular way of eating, not surprisingly, the weight returned. Still, Brenner thinks that if you can stick to the regimen, at the least, your ability to enjoy healthy foods and their natural flavors will increase. "I don't know if the Shangri-La Diet is the answer to all the factors that contribute to overeating and weight gain," she reflected, "but I do know that when I followed the technique, I lost weight."[5]

What does focusing on flavors in food suggest about food, eating, and your weight? It tells us that food, in part, is a function of its flavors and that when you take the time to savor flavors and truly taste all elements of your meal, an invisible, but soul-satisfying dynamic somehow manifests that is truly nourishing. The sensory disregard part of this eating style says that you don't have to solve all aspects of your relationship to food to achieve and maintain a normal weight: you can lower the odds of overeating and weight gain just by focusing on the flavors in your food. Roberts's "flavor theory" also confirms the problems inherent in the food fretting eating style, which includes traditional dieting based on a prescribed food regimen. Even if, as Roberts states, he's not suggesting a traditional diet, what he is proposing is still . . . well . . . a diet. And, as Brenner experienced when she went off the oil or sugar-water regimen, her time-tested eating habits and weight returned. If we take a closer look at the "transcendent" eating experience she had while focusing on flavors, we can get a better sense of the "spiritual disconnection" half of this eating style, and how you can use it to your advantage to overcome overeating.

By listening to this invisible mind-body message in your meals, you're likely to replace eating on autopilot with the amount of food your body really needs. Isn't it amazing? Simply by focusing on the flavors in your food, you may lower the odds of overeating and weight gain.

Meals of Mystery and Meaning

I vividly remember the moment I was introduced to the idea that a spiritual, meaningful connection to food has been integral to humankind for millennia. I was in New Delhi, India, where I had been invited to give a workshop at the First International Conference on Lifestyle and Health. During a discussion I had with Hindu cardiologist Dr. K. L. Chopra, father and mentor of the well-known author Deepak Chopra, he told me that the *Bhagavad Gita*, Hindu scripture, presents *prana*, the vital life force of the universe, as a cosmic consciousness that is metabolized when we eat. When you cook, you transfer your emotions into the food; in turn, when you eat the food, you metabolize the consciousness, or *prana*, with which the food was prepared.

Fascinated by the possibility that consciousness could alter the food we eat, I began a search to unearth wisdom about the profound meaning of food in our lives, to examine food and eating in the light of spiritual sustenance, to explore the interconnectedness between human consciousness and food. What I discovered is that most worldviews have been lush for millennia with sacred symbolism and spiritual beliefs surrounding food.

For instance, food was considered hallowed by the early Israelites, a means to worship Allah by Muslims, and a medium for transmitting psychic substance between individuals by Hindus. In the Christian community, the Eucharist (from the Greek *eucharisto*, meaning "to give thanks") uses bread and wine to connect to deeper mysteries. "We cannot see the secret vital force . . . which gives life to the grape and the grain," wrote mystic and nun Hildegard of Bingen in the twelfth century. "Yet the same force is at work when the bread and wine of the Eucharist are transformed into the flesh and blood of Christ."[6]

Though it is usually only a bite of bread and a swallow of wine (or juice) that contemporary Christians consume when they receive the Eucharist (or take Communion), the meal is rich in many ways—as is the Enlightened Diet, which is proposing a whole person nutrition program that feeds each aspect of our being. Such multidimensional nourishment is present when participants partaking of the Eucharist are fed physically with bread and beverage, nourished emotionally by being part of something holy, filled spiritually by experiencing Jesus' godliness, and satisfied socially through sharing sustenance with others.

The belief that a divine power could be ingested has its roots in early Pagans, who practiced a ritual of sacrifice wherein they actually ingested parts of the body of an animal that represented a certain god. When Jesus took bread and wine, blessed it, and said, "This is my body" and "This is my blood . . . which is to be poured out for many," he was walking the well-trodden path of those earlier pre-Christian sacrificial rites. Indeed, he was pursuing and obtaining spiritual sustenance through a profoundly meaningful, superconscious awareness of, and connection to, the mystery of life inherent in humans and in the nourishment that is food.

Filling the Void

In chapter 4, "Emotional Eating," when I was discussing Barbara Birsinger's research on emotional eating, I told you about the difference between having a nutritional craving for protein or carbohydrates, for example, versus a craving that is based on emotions that are often uncomfortable and unpleasant, such as loneliness, anger, or anxiety. In the sensory disregard eating style, we aren't addressing emotions;

we're alluding to a deep, internal hunger for something more intangible than food. Often, that "something more" is a profound yearning for spiritual sustenance; a longing to fill that empty feeling and lack of meaning and purpose in our lives; and a need to have a deeper connection with ourselves and others, indeed, the world. Aware of the spiritual element of overeating, Birsinger invited the Reverend Josephine Smith to work with the participants in the study by helping them feel more spiritually fulfilled through meditation, prayer, and spiritual community. If someone in the group needed to talk during the session, Smith was available to work with that person one on one.

What is especially intriguing about Birsinger's program is that spiritual connection is so integral that she called it "Conversations with Bod: Discovering the Spiritual Archetypal and Symbolic Messages in Food, Eating, Body Language, and Weight." Her rationale: longtime food restrictors or those who live their lives on a restriction-bingeing cycle, need to get in touch with their own biology again. "There's a disconnection from the body," Birsinger says, "a disconnect at the neck. The more severe the eating disorder, the more severe is the disconnection. Once a person gets to this point, a structured, regular eating plan is needed so the body can be reminded again about what it feels like to be hungry or full. Once they can feel and sense their internal hunger and satiety signals, they're able to learn and implement Intuitive Eating and get well."[7]

Birsinger helps people fill a spiritual void by showing them how to "shift focus from the external world around eating to an internal one," in other words, by becoming aware of why we make the food choices we do. The next step is to learn that the food choices we make have an important purpose; this gives people a sense of acceptance and compassion for themselves regarding their eating habits and behaviors. The big shift, she says, "is realizing how food has been serving as a way to take care of yourself. Once people get this, it's an epiphany; they realize that can change. And when this happens, it leads to optimal eating and weight loss."[8]

Sensory Regard Strategies

We've already discussed what it means to "eat with your senses" by taking in, for example, the color, textures, and aromas of food. But did you know that while there are five key senses (sight, smell, touch, taste, and motion or movement—or kinesthetic response), for millennia, Eastern healing systems, such as India's Ayurveda, traditional Chinese medicine (TCM), and Tibetan Medicine, have turned to six flavors in food to signal optimal eating and complete nutrition? I had been familiar with the role of the six tastes in Ayurveda and TCM, but I discovered its place in Tibetan Medicine during a lecture by Tibetan physician Dr. Namgyal Qusar. In response to a question from a member of the audience about optimal food preparation and nutrient preservation, Dr. Qusar responded by clarifying the Tibetan concept of "balance," consuming food from all food groups—both plant- and animal-based. Then, he added that for complete nutrition, you have to eat all six tastes: sweet, sour, salty, bitter, pungent, and astringent. In other words, Tibetan nutrition uses a finely honed sense of taste to ascertain whether a meal is balanced, and to find out, you have to focus your attention on the flavors inside your mouth as you chew.[9] The six tastes are so integral to health and well-being in Ayurveda that some ancient Ayurvedic schools encourage a sequence of tastes in a meal that progresses from sweet to salty, sour, pungent, bitter, and then astringent.

Savor six tastes. To put the concept of the six tastes into practice, gather the ingredients to make the unique Thai appetizer salad called *miang kam* (described earlier in this chapter): one each lime, small red onion, and red pepper; a piece of ginger; two tablespoons of roasted coconut; some honey (perhaps ¼ cup); and about ten spinach leaves. Except for the spinach, chop each food into tiny pieces. Next, spread a thin layer of honey (perhaps a teaspoon) on one spinach leaf, then take a pinch of each ingredient and sprinkle it over the sticky honey. Now, roll up the spinach leaf, creating a small food-filled tube. With your eyes closed, take a bite and begin to chew. Focus solely on the food in your mouth. Can you taste fantastic flavors? Are you able to identify one or more of the six tastes? Simply appreciate every single flavor.

Engage your senses. Experiencing food with your senses can connect you to the sacred, to the mystery of life, to other beings (indeed, to "being"). It's possible for you to nourish yourself this way with one of humankind's most simple and basic foods—bread— whether you're having a sandwich with friends, buttering bread at a restaurant, or having friends or family members over to create communion by sharing bread, cheese, and fruit, in your home.

Making such a meaningful connection calls for engaging all your senses: sight, touch, smell, taste, and hearing. To do this, *look* at the bread you are going to eat and become aware of its texture and color. Is it smooth, rough, light, or dark? When you take the bread in your hands, what does it *feel* like? Is it soft, tough, or grainy? Next, identify the *smell* of the bread. Is it sweet? Sour? Or in between? When you take a bite of the bread, do you *taste* one or more flavors? (Hint: the taste of food often changes as you chew.) Finally, how does the bread you're chewing *sound*? Loud or subtle?

Each time you break bread is an opportunity to be nourished spiritually. But . . . the extent to which this connection is revealed to you depends on your heartfelt intention and the degree to which you are willing to infuse bread (and all food and eating) with the mystery of sensory regard.

Connection Strategies

The antidote to sensory disregard and spiritual disconnection is discovering how to "eat from a place of spirit." A phrase coined by clinical psychologist Michael Mayer, it means that when you eat, you access *chi*, a centuries-old concept from China that describes the lifeforce within all living things, from feelings to food. When you cultivate *chi*, "you merge with the mysterious energy source in the world that is life itself," says Mayer. And, because such a comprehensive connection soothes the soul, it holds the power to fill the sense of emptiness that drives many of us to overeat.[10]

Earlier in this chapter, I told you about Judaism's havdalah ceremony, which captures the senses as a reminder to hold on to the Sabbath's moments of sweetness and peace during the busy work week. Bringing similar attention and regard to food and eating and the entire experience of dining means you're eating *from* the heart. When you do, this might be described in Hebrew as *yetzirah*, the spiritual awareness of unity and connection. And it is this understanding, recognition, and perception that fills and nourishes heart and soul.

Eat like a yogi. Devout yogis—people who practice yoga—follow a philosophy of *Sanatana dharma*, the Sanskrit expression for the underlying, eternal, true essence of all life. Such a philosophy complements the *Bhagavad Gita*, which encourages honoring all living things—including food—as part of an interdependent oneness. Approached with such a focus, the consciousness, or mentality, you bring to food may be the most important ingredient in the meal. When preparing or cooking food, think positive, loving, appreciative thoughts. After all, such a mentality may be transferred into the food, enhance digestion, and empower the food with the ability to nourish body, mind, and soul.

Like vitamins and minerals in life-giving foods, negative, angry thoughts are believed to be metabolized, too. Because of this, do not eat when you're angry, because negative thoughts are believed to create toxins that eventually are secreted by the glands. Also, anger or stress may limit the production of digestive enzymes in our stomachs, making it difficult for food to be adequately digested (see chapter 7, "Unappetizing Atmosphere," for more about this).

Brahman is the Sanskrit word that attempts to describe the indescribable; "a supreme, blissful consciousness" only hints at its meaning. Such a noble frame of mind is believed to contribute to optimal digestion. Just before eating, meditate on the following verse from the *Bhagavad Gita* (4:24), which express *Brahman* this way:

The process of eating is Brahman;
>The offering [of food] is Brahman.
The person offering is Brahman,
>And the fire is also Brahman.
Thus by seeing Brahman everywhere in action,
>He [alone] reaches Brahman.

Experience a Eucharist consciousness. Most religions and cultures intuitively have developed rituals that use food as a vehicle to connect to their deeper significance. For instance, believed to transform (either literally or symbolically, depending on the denomination) the bread and wine of the Sacrament into Jesus' body and blood, Communion provides an opportunity for believers to experience a profound spiritual connection through food. In part, the path includes connecting to the Divine here on earth through a ritual that engages all your senses: sight, hearing, touch, smell, and taste.

Spiritual connection may manifest in other ways. During the Thanksgiving holiday, millions of Americans gather together to share a meal of thanks with family and friends. As we consume the lavish meal of turkey and dressing, potatoes, cranberries, and pumpkin pie, we are honoring, and connecting with, the harvest of 1621, when about fifty settlers at the Plymouth Plantation invited approximately one hundred neighboring Native Americans to celebrate a much-appreciated crop of corn, barley, and peas. After all, these were friends who had helped them through hard times. Imagine the gratitude they held in their hearts during this meal!

Make each meal meaningful. As with my friend Keri Brenner's transcendent dining experience, the aesthetics of tea mind, the scents of the Sabbath, living a Eucharist consciousness, and Larry's special birthday celebration at Statholdergaarden, it's possible to make each meal a feast for both the senses and the soul. Accomplishing this calls for "charging the *chi*" by approaching food from that "place of spirit." When you eat with such heartfelt regard, you open the door to feeling connected to yourself and others, indeed, to the entire universe. At the same time, as you become more and more connected to your true nature, you make it more and more possible for your natural, normal weight to manifest.

Grow your own food. Gardening and growing the food that you cook creates a strong connection among you, the land, and the seasons. If you don't have space to garden, consider growing your own windowsill herb garden. Or buy food from your local farmers' market to experience the sensual pleasures of sampling and buying fresh, seasonal food; at the same time, you'll get to meet and appreciate the people who grow or make it.

Overcoming Sensory Disregard

With this discussion of sensory disregard, we have revealed the spiritual ingredient of the Enlightened Diet, that is, to savor flavors when you eat, and to take the time to create a meaningful connection to the food before you by appreciating all that went into bringing the food to you.

Our research on the seven eating styles highlights the mistake many make in thinking about food, eating, and weight loss, which is the basic belief that a simple formula—eat less, move more—will cure the problem. Such a conviction, though, underestimates the complexity of people's food choices and eating behaviors. Each eating style that makes up the Enlightened Diet and our whole person nutrition program for nourishing your biological, psychological, spiritual, and social well-being reveals that we overeat and we're overweight for many reasons: too much dieting (food fretting), distraction while eating (task snacking), unpleasant feelings (emotional eating), denatured fake food (fast foodism), isolated eating (solo dining), an unsettling environment (unpleasant atmosphere), and a sensory and spiritual vacuum or spiritual disconnection (sensory disregard). In other words, our research reveals that there are many reasons so many of us find it so hard to *eat less* and that, realistically, we have many biological, psychological, spiritual, and social reasons to *eat more.*

So far, each chapter on the eating styles has identified personal food, eating, and weight-related challenges, while shedding light on the science that supports the Rx for each eating style. At the same time, we've given you step-by-step strategies for creating your own whole person nutrition plan based on your individual needs and your personal nutrition and health goals. The next chapter, "Enlightened Exercise," shows you some similarities between the Enlightened Diet and the multidimensional benefits that movement and motion can bring to your biological, psychological, spiritual, and social well-being. As you'll see, Enlightened Exercise enhances the Enlightened Diet because it is a whole person exercise partner that helps you achieve and maintain your optimal weight.

Chapter 9

Enlightened Exercise

You may recall that in the first chapter of this book, I described the Enlightened Diet as a way of life, a "whole person" approach to nutrition and eating that nourishes your biological, psychological, spiritual, and social well-being. If your intention is to lose weight, I wrote, and you stay with it, you'll accomplish this . . . and much more: you'll also reap the rewards of more balanced emotions, spiritual well-being, and social connection. I call these multidimensional ways in which the Enlightened Diet heals whole person nutrition because not only is this entire book about optimal eating strategies for weight loss, but it also shows you how to make the most of your meals so "all of you" will be nourished each time you eat.

So, too, with motion. Look up the word *motion*, and you'll find "movement," "action," and "activity" to describe it. Or "exercise," "training," and "workout." Whichever way you turn the kinetic kaleidoscope, as with the Enlightened Diet, exercise, too, heals you physically, emotionally, spiritually, and socially. And by burning calories and speeding up your metabolism, it also helps you stay slim. Because motion and movement have the power to heal multidimensionally, as do the antidotes to the seven eating styles discussed throughout this book (see chapter 10, "In Action," for more about putting the Enlightened Diet into action each day), I am including a chapter about what I describe as "enlightened exercise." How does enlightened exercise differ from more traditional exercise? As with the Enlightened Diet, the answer is both simple and profound: through an understanding and appreciation of how motion and movement impact your entire being.

Whole Person Exercise

Not long ago a friend named Bruce Heller told me how his passion for movement began: "It became part of my life when I began to ride my bike to school when I was in elementary school. By biking to school, to after-school activities, and to friends' homes, or to just hang out, I wasn't dependent on my parents to drive me places, so over time, riding my bike came to symbolize a sense of freedom and independence. When I was a teenager, I started to ride my bicycle with other kids in the neighborhood. Now, as an adult, I ride my mountain bike as a stress-relieving activity; I do it for hours as a way to relax and stay in shape."

Today, Heller is a family physician who is passionate about food and nutrition, exercise, and health. A specialist in Integrative Medicine who uses Western and Eastern healing practices to prevent and treat obesity and related ailments, ranging from heart disease and high blood pressure to diabetes, Heller first looks at lifestyle interventions to help his patients. And exercise plays a central role because not only does it influence his patients' physiology, helping them to prevent and reverse health conditions, but it also influences the mood, well-being, and overall vitality of a person. "We were made to move," says Heller. "Human beings evolved as moving animals."

Realizing that exercise holds the power to heal in every way, Heller integrates it into his holistic healing recommendations to patients; it is also an integral part of his own life, a way to balance the demands of a busy practice. During a recent conversation, Heller shared a particularly memorable enlightened exercise experience with me, one that took place while he was a medical resident, when he often worked one-hundred-hour weeks:

> I used to call Annadel State Park in Santa Rosa, California, my church. During residency when I was busy and sleep deprived, often the only time I would have for a major workout was Sunday mornings at Annadel. I would wake up anticipating my mountain bike ride. Because my life was so busy and I had so little time, taking off on my bike brought back the sense of freedom and independence I had experienced as a youth on my bicycle. But now bike rides are even more meaningful for me because they are augmented by my appreciation of the beauty of nature, which has always been where I go to recharge. Now, I look forward not only to moving my body, but also to being outside in a beautiful place surrounded by nature. For me, pine trees represent cathedral spires, and there is a contemplative quality to a redwood forest; this is quite a contrast to the hours I spent indoors when I was a resident, working long, late hours in a busy hospital, caring for sick people, often surrounded by life or death situations.
>
> To balance this, I would start Sunday mornings with a cup of tea, and gentle yoga, stretching and focusing on each position (*asana*) consciously and mindfully. Interestingly, even when you just anticipate exercise, your body prepares you for the activity you're about to engage in; your physiology changes in anticipation of exercise. Even before you start running or biking or doing the activity, blood vessels dilate to bring more blood to the muscles; your heart rate speeds up to increase cardiac output; and breathing rate increases. It's almost as if you're warming up without actually warming up. Most people think exercise is purely physical, but there's also a mind-body connection. Your body knows it's going to need more blood and oxygen to power the muscles you'll be using when you move, so it starts helping you out even before you actually begin.

Annadel is a 5,200-acre park, filled with creeks, redwood groves, and meadows, and has about forty miles of trails. Entering the park on a fire road, I would ride past children and their families who were picnicking and feeding ducks, while others would be fishing in a stock pond. The higher up in elevation I would go on my mountain bike, the narrower the dirt trails would become. I especially enjoyed this because these are the most technically challenging trails: you have to be careful to avoid rocks, ruts, and roots. When I ride up and down steep inclines and declines, it gives me a strong sense of well-being and accomplishment. With a sigh of relief, I appreciate that I made it to the top. My body feels good. When I'm riding my bike, focused and concentrating on the terrain in front of me, I'm not always able to appreciate nature. But now, at the top of the ridge, it's all around me. Now I can see it all at my leisure; I'm on top of the world.

But there's more. After riding through the pine forest in the park, and then up and down two steep peaks, Heller would often reward himself toward the end of the ride with a swim in the park's lake. The total time for his exercise experience was two, sometimes three, hours.

Physical Feats

When Heller started his ride, at the outset, he could sense which muscles were sore, and any stiffness in his legs or neck. But after twenty minutes on his bike, with his blood flowing, and his muscles warming, he hit his natural pace. At this stage of his ride, the terrain was still pretty mellow, with gently rolling hills. After about twenty-five minutes, he would get to his first steep incline, which meant about a mile and a half of uphill riding. To ease resistance, he would click into a lower gear, stand up on the pedals, and start working a lot harder to stay at the same speed or cadence (how fast you're spinning the pedals). His breathing would quicken, his heart would beat faster, and he would break a sweat. After about twenty minutes, he would get to the top of the hill.

Throughout the ride, Heller's body would automatically do what's necessary to give him energy for the activity: his blood vessels would dilate to bring more blood, a carrier of oxygen, to power his cells and energize his muscles. "The metabolism of your cells is like an engine," he explains. "You can be more efficient or less efficient at burning energy. If you don't exercise, and you're a couch potato, your body isn't doing what it is meant to do: move. Breathing and digesting food still take energy, but your engine is running idly and inefficiently."

In contrast, every time you exercise, you have a whole body experience for your cardiovascular, musculoskeletal, respiratory, endocrine, hematologic, neurologic, and psychologic systems. You burn calories (energy) and your metabolism speeds up, you stay limber and flexible, and you build your bone density. "You burn sugar (glucose), the fuel your body uses, just the way an engine uses gasoline," adds Heller. "This is especially important for diabetics, because when they exercise, their muscles use up glucose so it no longer stays in their bloodstream."

Move and be in motion for at least thirty minutes, five times a week, and you'll realize health benefits, including weight loss. And the benefits are ongoing: even while you're watching TV, aerobic training speeds up metabolism and burns calories. "It will make your metabolic engine run more efficiently, and burn more oxygen, which ultimately burns more glucose and allows you to lose weight," clarifies Heller.[1]

The Heart of Motion

Although many of us think of Integrative Medicine as the first whole person approach to health and healing in Western medicine, Naturopathic Medicine (sometimes called "Naturopathy") has offered a comprehensive approach to health and healing since it evolved thousands of years ago as an effective medicine to treat diseases. Indeed, with his teaching that "nature is healer of all diseases," the Greek physician Hippocrates (c. 460 BCE–c. 370 BCE), who is often referred to as "the father of medicine" in recognition of his lasting contributions to the field, is thought to be the earliest naturopathic physician.

Today, modern naturopathic physicians (NDs) continue to offer a comprehensive system of health care based on the principle that the body tends toward health if you live according to the basic principles that govern human life—and one of those principles is keeping the body in motion. "Every molecule, cell, tissue, and organ has a purpose," naturopathic physician Bruce Milliman told me. "All systems are geared to be engaged according to nature's design. For the natural forces of health and healing to be optimized—in muscles or joints or the brain or nervous system or blood and lymph systems or in bone and cartilage or any organ system—you have to use it or lose it.'"

Indeed, the five natural elements of Milliman's "hierarchy of necessities to live" include air, water, sleep, food, and physical activity. During my conversation with Milliman, it was the element of physical activity that particularly caught my attention, because of the unique perspective he brings to it. "We have two circulatory systems," he explained. The first and primary one, the *circulatory system*—the one with which most of us are familiar—includes the heart, veins, arteries, and blood vessels. The *lymphatic system* parallels the circulatory system, Milliman explained, but unlike the circulatory system, it does not have a heart. Instead, the heart of this second circulatory system is *physical activity, motion*, and *movement*. And it functions almost exclusively by the moving of your limbs—your arms and legs. Consider walking. When you walk, for example, the motion of going up and down causes the lymphatic fluids in your body to move up and down within the lymphatic system; in turn, this helps your muscles contract each time you move your limbs. And all this is happening in unison with your breathing, while your diaphragm moves up and down. And as it moves, it compresses the lymphatic system, which has little valves that allow the lymph fluid to flow.

Which brings us to Milliman's second key concept (use it or lose it was the first)—what he calls the Black Box Theory: stuff in equals stuff out plus stuff stored. It's all about input and output. "Physical activity is an output," Milliman clarifies. It also integrates and balances the forces of the "use it or lose it" principle. Put another way, because physical activity is an expression of how fit you are, it determines the degree of freedom you have in your life to be healthy and to function autonomously. When you're not fit, and if you're taking in more energy than you put out, it's likely to take different forms, such as accumulated fat, or arthritis, or swelling (edema). The concept is simple: if you don't do what you need to do (meaning, you don't do some form of motion and movement on a regular basis), your circulatory (blood) and lymphatic (lymph) systems won't function optimally; this, in turn, increases the odds that you'll gain weight or develop some other ailment. Motion and your physical well-being: it's all interconnected, as is exercise and your emotional well-being.[2]

Of Movement, Moods, and Weight

When bicyclist and physician Bruce Heller is in good shape, he welcomes the challenge of riding up steep inclines. In Annadel State Park, the trails range from gentle and rolling, to shorter, rocky sections with steep ascents and descents. "I loved the challenge of steep and rutted trails, and trying to stay upright while going up a steep incline," he told me.

> Not only is it a great cardiovascular challenge, but it's also a technical challenge because I have to choose a line (a term used by skiers to describe planning a path to follow) and keep my balance. Then I would feel exhilarated going downhill fast, quite a contrast to cruising through the flat redwood groves at the bottom, where it is super quiet because the abundant redwood duff on the forest floor absorbs sounds.

During the challenge of riding up and down the first steep hill, I'm concentrating on what I'm doing, and I'm completely focused on the task at hand. During this time, I'm filled with a sense of well-being; a strong feeling of accomplishment. The second major ascent and descent in the park is even steeper. As I get closer and closer to the top, I'm feeling more like I'm in the wilderness. There is no noise from cars, and I'm feeling like I've really gotten away from it all. When I get to the top, I may pause for some water or a snack. At the same time, I'm appreciating my surroundings, along with the coyotes, deer, and hawks that are often a part of it all.[3]

Exhilaration, well-being, accomplishment, appreciation: these aren't words we often associate with exercise. But if you exercise regularly, as Heller does, and you take the time to tune in to your emotions while you're in motion and when you stop, it's likely you'll be feeling pretty good. Ongoing exercise (thirty minutes or more) causes hormones (naturally occurring chemical messengers in your body) to kick in. And one of these key chemicals is endorphins. Produced in the pituitary gland, endorphins not only *decrease your appetite*, but they also reduce tension and anxiety. Make exercise a regular part of your life, and after several months, you'll experience a super-high from endorphins. And it gets better. They'll continue to circulate in your blood for quite a while after you've exercised.

While feel-good endorphins may lessen your appetite, other weight loss–related hormones are produced when you exercise regularly. These hormones include 17 beta estradiol, the most biologically active estrogen, which helps break down body fat stores so it can be used for fuel; testosterone, which increases your metabolism and decreases body fat; growth hormone, which increases the use of fat when you exercise; thyroxine (T4), a hormone made by the thyroid gland that increases your metabolic rate; and epinephrine, a hormone produced mostly in the adrenal medulla, which stimulates stored fat to break down.

You stand to gain even more benefits from exercise in addition to the runner's high that endorphins create and the fat-burning that other hormones produce. You may recall that in chapter 4, "Emotional Eating," I told you about emotional eaters, most of whom seek food in an attempt to manage unpleasant feelings, such as depression, anxiety, or anger. When negative emotions emerge, emotional eaters turn to food as a distraction, as a way to run away from, and to numb, these feelings. If you're a regular exerciser, the endorphins and other hormones you produce can replace food as your best friend when you're feeling blue. In other words, be in motion on a regular basis, and you'll be less likely to be an emotional eater. Endorphins do more than decrease your appetite: they also reduce tension and anxiety; in this way, they hold the power to replace depression and anxiety, and other unwelcome feelings, with a mild state of euphoria.

In the Zone

"Being 'in the zone' is an indescribable experience," Heller told me. "When playing Ultimate Frisbee, I used to describe my state of mind as 'relaxed attention.' During these times, my body would be doing exactly what I wanted it to do—without my being especially attentive or focusing on it. When this happens, I have a sense of being one with the motion and my surroundings, for instance, with the bike and the trail on which I'm riding. During these times, my body knows what to do. I'm not intentionally exercising; all motion and movement is flowing effortlessly."[4]

Many athletes describe Heller's experience of being "in the zone" in a similar way. Without conscious intention—or attention—their mind-body becomes one with the activity and environment. Somehow, they're not quite in their body anymore; there's a sense that they're one with their body and the environment—and even though they may be putting out a fair amount of energy, they have a sense of effortlessness. Could it be the endorphins that have kicked in, or the alpha brain waves that combat depression and put you in a state of relaxation? Or is it a mystery, the same life force that enhances digestion and somehow stabilizes your weight when you eat with sensory regard (see chapter 8, "Sensory Disregard," for insights into these ingredients) and in serene surroundings (see chapter 7, "Unappetizing Atmosphere" for more about connection to your environment)? "This spiritual connection—going in or out of the zone—can happen anytime," offers Heller. "There's no way to anticipate when this is going to happen."[5]

Often after his bike ride in Annadel State Park, while he's feeling gratified by a challenging workout, emotionally high from the endorphins, and in the zone, Heller would often jump into the park's lake, which is surrounded by trees, located in a bowl-like valley. He would end his ride by taking a quick dip to cool off. Swimming, looking at the blue sky, he would hang out for perhaps twenty or thirty minutes, savoring the last phase of his mountain biking adventure; the end of the ride . . . for now.

Social Fitness

When I first moved to San Francisco, the bus I took to my job in the financial district would pass through the city's large Chinatown district. As the bus descended the narrow, hilly, and shaded part of Sacramento Street, I would watch, transfixed, as a large group of people practiced tai chi (an ancient Chinese discipline that involves the mind, breath, and movement to create a calm, natural balance of energy) in silence each morning in an outdoor park in the cool morning fog. In unison and in super–slow motion, each person in the group would move through each ancient and exact movement and motion of his or her tai chi practice. Then, as now, the image seemed like an oasis, something not quite real that had the illusion of appearing suddenly and unexpectedly in the center of a major city.

Whether the activity is soccer, dance, hiking, football, bowling, or ancient Asian movements, for thousands of years people have exercised with others. As with social nutrition—dining with others instead of solo—physical activity has typically been practiced as a team activity. "I was part of the Ultimate Frisbee Team in college," Bruce Heller told me, "a group sport that is played on most college campuses. Club teams play in almost all major cities throughout the world: Europe, Africa, Asia. A lot of my friends that I made twenty or more years ago, when I played competitive Frisbee, are still some of my best friends now. After tournaments, we would always eat out, and share memories of the day. Then, as now, it's one of the most enjoyable ways to connect with others."[6]

Of Eating and Exercise

Clearly, both food and movement have the power to heal in multiple dimensions—physically, emotionally, spiritually, and socially. After all, as with the Enlightened Diet, doesn't enlightened exercise suggest that, like facets of a kaleidoscope that change with each turn of the tube, movement and motion influence your physical, emotional, spiritual, and social well-being, as well as your weight; in other words, your entire being? Isn't each facet a reflection of the other? Isn't each both independent and interdependent on the other?

The parallel between optimal eating and exercise and their power—when practiced in unison—to achieve and maintain optimal weight has been proven over and over again by studies on the topic. An especially intriguing one was conducted by researchers in the Department of Kinesiology at George Washington University Medical Center in Washington, DC. To find out whether diet, aerobic exercise, or diet plus exercise brought the most weight loss, they looked at *all* relevant studies reported in English, in peer-reviewed medical journals, during the past twenty-five years. Not surprisingly, diet plus exercise tended to be the superior program for obese adults to lose weight and keep it off.[7]

Enlightened Exercise Options

Our society has become very sedentary. Television, computers, and video games contribute to children's inactive lifestyles; indeed, 43 percent of adolescents watch more than two hours of television each day. Children, especially girls, become less active as they progress through adolescence. The antidote? Look over the menu of movement options I've created for you, then choose your own preferences for getting in motion, based on your personal inclinations and lifestyle.

Before you begin, though, I would like to suggest that you reread the "Stages of Change" section in chapter 2, "Food Fretting." If you recall, the Stages of Change give you insights into how to change successfully—for instance, from being a nonexerciser to making movement and motion a part of your everyday life—and specific strategies about how you can best help yourself in your effort to become a "successful loser." The mistake many of us make when we think of losing weight by modifying meals and exercise is ignorance of where we are in the Stages of Change cycle, which tells you whether you are ready, really, really ready, to change, or whether you would benefit by first contemplating your plan. By not jumping ahead to a stage for which you may not be ready, you increase your odds of making exercise an integral aspect of your everyday life. To get started, consider some of the options below. Look them over, then identify the activities you resonate with the most. Then think about when and how you can fit them into your life. Be realistic and compassionate with yourself. If you can fit in five or ten minutes, perhaps three times a day, to do something you enjoy, that's an accomplishment. "Extremercise," for hours at a time, isn't for everyone.

Follow Your "Fitness Instinct"

Medical anthropologist and fitness expert Peg Jordan has created a unique and personalized approach to working out. Her philosophy: make it something you love to do, and you're more likely to succeed. To help you figure this out, Jordan has developed workout options based on what she calls your "fitness instinct," that is, ways to move based on your personal, inborn preferences and personality. For instance, if you're a highly competitive businessperson, a stay-at-home, staid piece of equipment such as a treadmill is just going to gather dust. You're more likely to thrive playing raquetball three times a week with someone you can compete with aggressively. In contrast, Jordan offers the example of "a soccer mom who is other-directed, taking care of everybody." This person "needs to be on the buddy system for exercise," suggests Jordan, whose fitness philosophy is based on a research study. "Her best friend and she should walk together or she should have a buddy to do swing dancing with." Adds Jordan: "Exercise for this type should be social."

Living the Enlightened Diet

With this chapter on enlightened exercise, we have given you insights into enhancing the Enlightened Diet by expanding your vision of what a whole person approach to food, eating, and achieving optimal weight can be. With this chapter, we are suggesting that you also include whole person exercise options that feed you physically, emotionally, spiritually, and socially, each time you are in action. How can you put together each element of the Enlightened Diet that we have discussed throughout this book so that you can reap its rewards each day? The next chapter, "In Action," will give you step-by-step guidelines for optimal eating . . . all ways.

Peg Jordan's "Get-Going" Exercise Suggestions

Here are some of Jordan's ideas, based on four different categories of "mindset" and activities that match each one.

When you're tired . . .

Play with a hoola hoop.

Practice tai chi.

Take a yoga class.

When you're wired . . .

Do a walking meditation.

Move to music.

Get a massage.

When you're experiencing body boredom . . .

Take a salsa or swing-dancing class.

Take improvisational acting lessons.

Garden or build sand castles.

When you're stuck in routine . . .

Take a kick-boxing class.

Go river rafting.

Take a rigorous nature hike.[8]

Mix It Up

Here's a varied selection of movement and motion options.

Every Day

Park your car a few blocks away from your destination.

Take the stairs instead of the elevator.

Walk to the store or mailbox.

Three to Five Times per Week

Aerobic Exercise:

Walk briskly during your lunch break or after dinner.

Bicycle to and from work or on a stationary bicycle.

Take a dance class.

Recreation:

Practice a martial art, such as akido or karate.

Play basketball, softball, or baseball.

Try roller skating in your local park.

Two to Three Times per Week

Flexibility and Strength:

Stretch, or try yoga or Pilates.

Do push-ups, curl-ups, and sit-ups.

Lift weights.

Make an "In Motion" Plan

The United States Department of Agriculture (USDA) recommends that adults exercise at least thirty minutes daily; children and teens should target fifty minutes of activity each day. The USDA Physical Activity Pyramid offers both *moderate* and *vigorous* physical activity possibilities.

Moderate Physical Activities

Walking briskly (about $3\frac{1}{2}$ miles per hour)

Hiking

Gardening

Dancing

Golfing (walking and carrying clubs)

Bicycling

Weight training (a general light workout)

Vigorous Physical Activities

Running, jogging (5 miles per hour)

Bicycling (more than 10 miles per hour)

Swimming (freestyle laps)

Aerobics

Walking fast ($4\frac{1}{2}$ miles per hour)

Lifting heavy weights

Playing competitive basketball[9]

Chapter 10

In Action

Whenever I'm presenting, teaching, or lecturing about the Enlightened Diet and whole person nutrition, I often begin by inviting participants to share their recollection of an especially memorable meal. It is amazing that without fail people include all the ingredients of the Enlightened Diet. Always, the stories are filled with food-related pleasure, mindfulness, good feelings, fresh food and dining with others in a pleasant atmosphere. The memorable meals I hear about are never the seven eating styles in action: eating fast food, alone, to manage unpleasant feelings, while fretting about the high fat content, in a hectic, unpleasant atmosphere, while driving and talking on a cell phone, with no regard. While thinking about memorable meals and the Enlightened Diet, I was riveted to the TV when Mireille Guiliano, the French-born CEO of Clicquot, Inc., Veuve Clicquot's American subsidiary, and author of *French Women Don't Get Fat*, appeared on the *Oprah Winfrey Show* to tell her story. She came to the United States as a teenage exchange student, gained twenty pounds, then gained ten more pounds when she returned to France and continued her American-style way of eating.[1]

Guiliano's weight loss success starts with her rock bottom moment when she first returned to France. It had been a year since she'd seen her family when she descended from the SS *Rotterdam*, in the 1960s.

Expecting her beret-clad father's face to light up when he saw her, instead, he looked stunned. As she came closer, he continued to stare at her, and then, as her brother and American shipmate stood nearby, his first words to his beloved daughter were, *"Tu ressembles à un sac de patates"* ("You look like a bag of potatoes"). As hurtful as this comment was, it wasn't enough for her to take action to lose the twenty pounds she had gained while in the States. Instead, Guiliano continued her American eating habits while attending university in Paris, where she gained ten more pounds by Christmas. And then, during holiday break, at the urging of Guiliano's mother, Dr. Meyer, the kind, gentlemanly, family physician, whom Guiliano calls "Dr. Miracle," intervened. Losing the weight would be easy, he assured her, once she returned to the French way of eating.

After Guiliano kept a three-week record of what, how much, when, and where she ate, she realized she had adopted quite a few typically American eating styles; for instance, she ate while walking or standing (task snacking) and grabbing whatever was convenient and available (fast foodism). Permanent change, she realized with the help of Dr. Miracle, called for achieving equilibrium not only in her food choices, but also in all aspects of her life. To do this, *she would have to engage her mind.* During the next three months, Guiliano relearned the way of the French woman. And the weight came off. Guiliano is now in her fifties, and the weight has stayed off—without dieting and excessive exercise. Her secret to success? She reconnected to her country's fresh food culinary roots and its pleasurable approach to food, eating, and the aesthetics of dining. When I looked closely at some of Guiliano's comments to Oprah, clearly, how she did it is the Enlightened Diet in action, the antithesis of the seven eating styles linked with overeating, overweight, and obesity: food fretting, task snacking, emotional eating, fast foodism, solo dining, unpleasant atmosphere, and sensory disregard. For instance, she mentioned enjoying food and relating to it as a pleasure; eating chocolate or other sweets, but in small portions; not counting calories; not working on her computer when it's time for lunch; snacking on fresh, whole food; eating with friends; eating with her senses and paying attention to the food before her; and finally, perceiving what, how, where, and with whom she eats to be a lifestyle philosophy.

At the start of this book and also in chapter 6, "Solo Dining," when I told you about the Roseto and rabbit experiments, both of which imply there is a mystery to how we metabolize food beyond what is measurable, I mentioned a powerful comment by physician Deepak Chopra about the consciousness we bring to meals: "When you look at nutrition from a purely scientific point of view, there is no place for consciousness. And yet, consciousness could be one of the crucial determinants of the metabolism of food itself." Clearly, Chopra's comment addresses the power of both measurable nutrients in fresh food and harder-to-measure nutrients that seem to protect our weight and well-being when we eat filled with pleasure, mindfulness, feel-good feelings, social support, aesthetic awareness, and sensory delight—the ingredients that make up the Enlightened Diet. Guiliano might describe this as having to engage her mind if she were to be successful at losing weight. Chopra's comment resonates with me because, at its core, it encompasses each of the biological, psycho-logical, spiritual, and social elements of the Enlightened Diet that are inherent in whole person nutrition *and* nourishment.

I am asking you to consider Chopra's insight in light of the Enlight-ened Diet because the antidotes to each eating style I have told you about throughout this book ask you to focus your attention on more, much more, than calorie counting, weight watching, fat grams, and carb content of food. Rather, the studies and stories I have told you about for each of the eating styles suggest that both the intentional and the unin-tentional awareness you bring to meals impacts the ways in which your mind and body use nutrients and calories and, in turn, impact your weight. Call it awareness, realization, or perception, the "consciousness" to which Chopra alludes suggests a special sensibility or sensitivity—an invisible, hard-to-measure mystery—that somehow plays an essential and critical role in the metabolism of food itself. As we've seen, when this consciousness is activated, it holds the power to end emotional eating, turn dietary deprivation into dietary delight, neutralize potentially artery-clogging cholesterol and fat you may have consumed, and also help Frenchwoman Mireille Guiliano stay slim for life.

What is it about the Enlightened Diet that brings so many benefits? Some time ago, an acquaintance gave me a key to what I believe is the answer. "My brother married a Frenchwoman, and he, his wife, and two small children live on the outskirts of Paris," he told me. "When I visited my six-year-old nephew at school, I noticed that he and his classmates were served a warm, full-course lunch on glass plates, which they ate while sitting around a small table, chatting with each other." I thought about this conversation when our research on whole person nutrition revealed the seven eating styles. Wasn't my friend, in essence, describing the Enlightened Diet? Our weight loss message comes down to this: eat flavor-filled fresh food, be aware of dining accoutrements, dine with others, savor every bite, and relax; in other words, each time you eat, embrace food as if you were following the Enlightened Diet. And eat this way from childhood through adulthood.[2]

Elemental Overview

The ultimate antidote to weight gain and related ailments is to live the Enlightened Diet each day. For many of you, this calls for *changing your relationship to food and eating*—biologically (eat fresh whole foods and don't diet), emotionally (eat for pleasure), spiritually (eat mindfully, with an aesthetic awareness), and socially (dine with others). As many of you realize by now, the Enlightened Diet reframes optimal nourishment as an eating practice for the whole person—and for a lifetime. However, reading about the Enlightened Diet, by itself, won't change what and how you eat, nor will it open the door to multidimensional nourishment and optimal weight. Rather, reaping the rewards of the

Enlightened Diet calls for implementing the antidotes to each eating style on a daily basis. It's not theory, it's not wishful thinking; it's about being proactive, taking action, and making your commitment to changing your relationship to food. To reap the rewards *now*, here is an overview of the seven elements—the key principles—of the Enlightened Diet. Look them over carefully, and familiarize yourself with them. Having an intimate understanding of each one is pivotal to overcoming overeating, overweight, and obesity.

THE ENLIGHTENED DIET
Antidotes to the Seven Eating Styles

Here are the elements of the Enlightened Diet, the essential antidote to each of the seven eating styles we've discussed throughout this book.

- **Food Fretting Rx:** Perceive food and the experience of eating as a social, ceremonial, sensual pleasure.
- **Task Snacking Rx:** Bring moment-to-moment non-judgmental awareness to each aspect of the meal.
- **Emotional Eating Rx:** Eat only for pleasure and when you're feeling feel-good feelings.
- **Fast Foodism Rx:** Choose fresh whole food in its natural state as often as possible.
- **Solo Dining Rx:** Share food-related experiences with others.
- **Unappetizing Atmosphere Rx:** Dine in psychologically and aesthetically pleasing surroundings.
- **Sensory Disregard Rx:** Savor flavors when you eat.

Each time you eat or participate in any food-related activity, remember that all seven elements of the Enlightened Diet count and that optimal nourishment includes both the familiar nutrients in food, as well as the psychological, spiritual, and social nutrients missing from the food charts. We created the elements of the Enlightened Diet to make it easy for you to practice them daily. For only by actually doing them each day will you be empowered to nourish your physical health, your emotions, your senses, and your social well-being. Also, be patient with yourself: making such sweeping changes in what, how, where, and even with whom you eat is a process. In other words, changing your relationship to food and overcoming overeating so that you may stay slim for life isn't likely to happen overnight: success takes ongoing nurturing, care, and regard . . . for yourself.

To enhance your odds for success and nutritional self-care, the following section gives you strategies for overcoming obstacles that may be keeping you from integrating the elements of the Enlightened Diet into your life.

Identifying Your Obstacles

At the beginning of this book, you filled out the What's Your Eating Style? profile. Needless to say, every person's profile is different. So, too, are the areas—and degrees—of resistance that some of you may experience in implementing the elements of the Enlightened Diet and getting the results you want—or don't want. In the profile, you identified the elements that are challenging for you, and others you already do easily and effortlessly. Look over the eating styles you pinpointed as being integral aspects of your food life and therefore hardest for you to overcome, then identify them below to discover strategies for moving closer to your biological, psychological, spiritual, and social nutrition goals.

Food Fretting

Obstacle: You perceive food and the experience of eating as a social, ceremonial, sensual pleasure, but you continue to be overly concerned about food, calories, and diets.

Strategy: Because so many of us have been taught that food fretting and obsessing about calories, weight, and dieting is normal, this eating style can be particularly challenging to turn around. But it is possible—if you decide to go against the dieting and deprivation norm and, instead, change your relationship to food and eating at the core. Doing this calls for nothing less than turning diet-think into pleasure-think, each time you eat. Each time you find yourself heading back on the calorie-counting roller coaster, halt the thought by closing your eyes, inhaling deeply, then exhaling as you release the thought and the related tension that surrounds it. Now, think of food and eating as one of life's greatest gifts . . . and pleasures.

Task Snacking

Obstacle: You bring moment-to-moment nonjudgmental awareness to each aspect of the meal, but you find it difficult to keep focused.

Strategy: It's natural and normal for thoughts to wander. That's why mindfulness meditation is called a practice; it's something you can practice for a lifetime. Here are three steps for bringing mindfulness to all food-related activities—from planning the meal to eating and washing dishes afterward. First, decide to focus on food and eating (or shopping or prepping, and so on). Simply become aware that you intend to do this. Second, if you find your attention wandering, gently let go of the thoughts or actions that are interfering with your intention and commitment and then refocus on food. Third, hold your intention and commitment to mindfulness and focus your attention on the food or food-related activity.

Emotional Eating

Obstacle: You eat only for pleasure and when you're feeling feel-good feelings, but your food cravings and negative emotions take over, making checking in difficult.

Strategy: Accessing the potent power that food has on your feelings—and vice versa—isn't always easy. In fact, our research on the seven eating styles revealed that emotions are more strongly related to overeating than any other element of the Enlightened Diet. The antidote: tease out the emotions that manifest before, during, and after you eat; this requires a subtle refocusing of attention—a shift of mind and heart, a new way of communicating with both yourself and your food. To accomplish this shift, prior to eating, set aside some specific time to observe and acknowledge your feelings without judgment or the impulse to act upon them. Simply *be* with your feelings, even if they're negative ones, even if it's uncomfortable for you.

Fast Foodism

Obstacle: You choose fresh whole foods in its natural state as often as possible, but the carrot cake is often more tempting than the carrot.

Strategy: Keep in mind that the optimal food guideline isn't about rigid dietary dogma, or rules and regulations; this is why we've qualified this guideline with the phrase "as often as possible." Our intention is to help you think of a variety of fresh, whole food as your most-of-the-time way of eating, not as yet another diet to follow for a while before returning to your usual way of eating. If you've accomplished this, congratulate yourself, and enjoy nonwhole food if you choose it intentionally and it is no longer typical for you. On the other hand, if you want something sweet and you also want to keep it fresh and whole, consider dates, figs, or a homemade fruit smoothie.

Solo Dining

Obstacle: You share food-related experiences with others, but you eat alone more often than not.

Strategy: If you often dine by yourself, the easiest way to change that is to bring others to your table through memory and by reflecting on past meals you shared with people you like. As you eat and think of prior dining experiences with others, consider what made the meals so memorable. Was it the people? The food? The atmosphere? The conversation? A special holiday or celebration? An outdoor picnic or an impromptu indoor meal? Once you identify the delightful elements of the shared meal, create a comparable dining event with friends, family members, or coworkers. Take pictures of the occasion, and place the photos of food and friends on your dining table; in this way, you can replicate the experience each time you eat.

Unappetizing Atmosphere

Obstacle: You would like to dine in psychologically and aesthetically pleasing surroundings, but you don't know where to begin.

Strategy: Both the psychological and the aesthetic surroundings in which you dine influence the meal in many ways. If you typically eat in an atmosphere that's fraught with fighting, hostility, or loud noises, here are some options for change. The most obvious action you can take is to change where you eat, or to stop dining with people who create an unpleasant atmosphere. If this isn't an option, ask others whether they can put their hostilities on hold while eating. Aesthetically, small changes can make a big difference: light some candles; play some favorite, soothing music; and use your best china. Make the atmosphere as pleasant as possible.

Sensory Disregard

Obstacle: You savor flavors when you eat, but you are finding it hard to make a meaningful connection to meals.

Strategy: Receiving meals with gratitude is the secret to savoring flavors in food; indeed, it's the secret to achieving all elements of the Enlightened Diet. To accomplish this, regard and acknowledge all aspects of the meal before you—from the nature that created it to the farmer who raised the crops. Identify at least one aspect of food to appreciate (for instance, nature and the elements, such as rain, earth, air, and sunshine). Perceive food (both plant- and animal-based) as an equal, in that it contains the mystery of life as do we human beings. As you eat, consider the alchemy, the interconnection, the oneness inherent in food and eating. Then, holding appreciation in your heart, focus on the flavors in the food. Make a brief blessing of appreciation: thank you for being.

Overcoming Obstacles

There are other steps you can take to break through obstacles that are keeping you from getting and staying on track with the Enlightened Diet. For instance, take a quick refresher course by rereading the chapters on the eating styles that are keeping you from being successful. Then, empower yourself to overcome any existing obstacle by doing this miniexercise.

1. Identify the eating style that is most challenging for you.
2. Write it down.
3. Identify the reasons you think it's hardest for you to do.
4. Create your own techniques for overcoming the obstacle you just identified.

Then there's the other side of success. For the eating styles you don't find challenging or that you don't resist, why do you think this is so? Which aspects of the Enlightened Diet resonate with you especially?

Moonlight Memory

"I'm thinking of charging everyone extra for the full moon and moonlight," announced chef Ruggero Gigli in his thick Italian accent from the outdoor porch of Villa Gigli, the combination restaurant and artist studio in Markleeville, California, owned by Gigli and his wife, Gina. A native of Florence, Gigli made the announcement to the approximately one hundred diners who were sitting, eating, and conversing at long tables in his restaurant's garden. He called the diners' attention to the resplendent moonlit setting just as we were about to embark on the first course of our meal: an exquisitely colored, perfectly flavored, textured, and scented pumpkin soup (*zuppa di zucca*). At Villa Gigli—indeed, throughout Italy, Europe, Asia, and worldwide—a first course is more, much more that a simple soup or starter: it is the beginning of the Enlightened Diet in action, it is the solution to the seven eating styles—food fretting, task snacking, emotional eating, fast foodism, solo dining, unappetizing atmosphere, and sensory disregard—we've discussed throughout this book, which lead to overeating, overweight, and obesity.

As Larry and I dined at Villa Gigli that magical evening, I couldn't help but realize how every aspect of the meal embodied the Enlightened Diet: we delighted in the entire experience; we focused on the food as we ate; we were filled with joy and gratitude; the food was exquisitely fresh; without distraction, we relished every aspect of the evening; we were dining with others in extraordinary surroundings; and we took the time to truly taste and savor our food.

A Taste for All Reasons

Throughout the Enlightened Diet, we have shown you how to eat optimally by revealing and demystifying each of the seven eating styles—the nutrients missing from the food charts. This new/ancient view asks that you pay attention to all of the eating styles each time you eat—and to understand and practice their antidotes every day. Ultimately, the message of the Enlightened Diet is simple: the healing gifts of food are available to you each time you eat. As a matter of fact, every time you shop for, prepare, and eat food you have the opportunity to live the Enlightened Diet. Along the way, you are empowering yourself to experience food as the symphonic masterpiece that it is, one that plays the notes of fresh food, positive feelings, in-the-moment mindfulness, culinary delight, pleasing surroundings, savory flavors, and social connection.

Weaving together the moments of a meal based on these elements also means you're creating conscious connection to *what* you're eating, *how* you're eating, and *with whom* you're eating. Creating the connection is not an easy task, for in our hurry-worry society, most of us no longer enjoy meals of fresh, whole food at the dining room table, filled with a sense of quietude, with people we love—that is, unless you're living the Enlightened Diet. When you eat from such a place of pleasure, you are fed more than food. Each dining experience becomes an occasion to nourish your entire being and to turn the tide of weight gain.

Taking pleasure in food, eating mindfully, nourishing yourself with positive emotions as you eat, savoring flavors and surroundings, eating with others, living and eating with an awareness of all aspects of the Enlightened Diet—all lie at the heart of achieving and maintaining optimal weight and well-being. Remember that it is a process, a lifetime adventure, one you can take to nourish your biological, psychological, spiritual, and social well-being each time you eat. In this way, each meal holds the potential to be a memorable meal.

Endnotes

Introduction: Ancient Food Wisdom Meets Modern Nutritional Science

1. Deepak Chopra, "Body, Mind and Soul," PBS, KQED-TV, San Francisco, March 7, 1995.

2. Deborah Kesten, *Feeding the Body, Nourishing the Soul* (Berkeley, CA: Conari Press, 1997).

3. Larry Dossey, *Reinventing Medicine: Beyond Mind-Body to a New Era of Healing* (New York: HarperCollins, 1999).

4. Deborah Kesten, *The Healing Secrets of Food* (Novato, CA: New World Library, 2001).

5. Deborah Kesten, "The Enlightened Diet: Integrating Biological, Spiritual, Social, and Psychological Nutrition," *Spirituality & Health* 4 (Winter 2003): 29–39; Deborah Kesten, "The Enlightened Diet Integrative Eating E-course," *Spirituality & Health* (December 16, 2002–January 24, 2003). Available at www.EnlightenedDiet.com.

6. David Riley, "Integrative Nutrition: Food's Multidimensional Power to Heal," *Explore: The Journal of Science and Healing* 1, no. 5 (September 2005): 341; Larry Scherwitz and Deborah Kesten, "Seven Eating Styles Linked with Overeating, Overweight and Obesity," *Explore: The Journal of Science and Healing* 1, no. 5 (September 2005): 340–41.

7. Riley, "Integrative Nutrition," 341.

Chapter 1: Whole Person Nutrition

1. Kenneth R. Pelletier, *The Best Alternative Medicine* (New York: Simon & Schuster, 2000).

2. Dossey, *Reinventing Medicine.*

3. All seven eating styles are statistically significant in terms of predicting overeating. Here is how they ranked, beginning with the strongest predictor: emotional eating (.561); food fretting (.318); fast foodism (.224); sensory disregard (.172); task snacking (.156); unappetizing atmosphere (.119); solo dining (-.028). The five statistically significant eating styles that predict overweight and obesity are: emotional eating (-.295); fast foodism (-.265); sensory disregard (-.068); task snacking (-.061); and unappetizing atmosphere (.057). This suggests that if a person typically practices all seven eating styles, she or he is likely to overeat; but practicing five of the eating styles is a strong predictor of becoming overweight or obese. Scherwitz and Kesten, "Seven Eating Styles Linked with Overeating, Overweight, and Obesity," 340-41.

Chapter 2: Food Fretting

1. K. M. Flegal, M. D. Carroll, R. J. Kuczmarski, and C. L. Johnson, "Overweight and Obesity in the United States: Prevalence and Trends," *International Journal of Obesity* 22 (1998): 39–47; A. H. Mokdad, M. K. Serdula, W. H. Dietz, et al., "The Spread of the Obesity Epidemic in the United States," *Journal of the American Medical Association* 282, no. 16 (1999): 1519–22.

2. B. M. Malinauskas, T. D. Raedeke, V. G. Aeby, and J. L. Smith, "Dieting Practices, Weight Perceptions, and Body Composition: A Comparison of Normal Weight, Overweight, and Obese College Females," *Nutrition Journal* 5, no. 11 (March 31, 2006), www.nutritionj.com/content/5/1/11 (accessed June 15, 2007);

M. K. Serdula, A. H. Mokdad, D. F. Williamson, et al., "Prevalence of Attempting Weight Loss and Strategies for Controlling Weight," *Journal of the American Medical Association* 282, no. 16 (1999): 1353–58.

3. G. D. Foster and T. A. Wadden, "What Is a Reasonable Weight Loss? Patients' Expectations and Evaluations of Obesity Treatment Outcomes," *Journal of Consulting and Clinical Psychology* 65, no. 1 (1997): 79–85; G. D. Foster, T. A. Wadden, S. Phelan, D. B. Sarwer, et al., "Obese Patients' Perceptions of Treatment Outcomes and the Factors That Influence Them," *Archives of Internal Medicine* 161, no. 17 (September 24, 2001): 2133–39.

4. R. Dalle Grave, S. Calugi, E. Molinari, M. L. Petroni, et al., "Weight Loss Expectations in Obese Patients and Treatment Attrition: An Observationsal Multicenter Study," *Obesity Research* 1311 (November 2005): 1961–69.

5. Tufts University, "Yes, but Is Weight Loss the Be-all and the End-all?" *Tufts Health & Nutrition Letter*, July 2004, www.healthletter.tufts.edu/issues/2004-07/weight.html (accessed June 15, 2007); Christopher D. Still, "Health Benefits of Modest Weight Loss—Penn State Geisinger Health Care System," Healthology, Inc., 2006, www.weightfocus.com (accessed March 16, 2006).

6. M. L. Dansinger, J. A. Gleason, J. L. Griffith, et al., "Comparison of the Atkins, Ornish, Weight Watchers, and Zone Diets for Weight Loss and Heart Disease Risk Reduction: A Randomized Trial," *Journal of the American Medical Association* 293, no. 1 (2005): 43–53; Daniel DeNoon, "4 Diets Face Off: Which Is the Winner? The Best Diet: The One You Stick With," WebMd Medical News, January 4, 2005, www.webmd.com (accessed July 24, 2006).

7. C. C. DiClemente and J. O. Prochaska, "Self Change and Therapy Change of Smoking Behavior: A Comparison of Processes of

Change in Cessation and Maintenance," *Addictive Behaviors* 89 (1982): 133–42; J. O. Prochaska and C. C. DiClemente, "Transtheoretical Therapy: Toward a More Integrative Model of Change," *Psychotherapy: Theory, Research and Practice* 19 (1982): 276–88.

8. Psychology Matters, APA Online, "Understanding How People Change Is First Step in Changing Unhealthy Behavior," www.psychologymatters.org/diclemente (accessed December 21, 2006); Robert Westermeyer, "A User-Friendly Model of Change," Habit Smart, September 5, 2005, www.habitsmart.com/ motivate.htm (accessed December 21, 2006).

9. *The American Heritage Dictionary of the English Language*, 4th ed. (New York: Houghton Mifflin, 2003).

Chapter 3: Task Snacking

1. CBS News, Healthwatch, "Car Cuisine: Food Industry Caters to Drivers Eating Behind the Wheel," November 9, 2005, www.cbsnews.com/stories/2005/11/09/health/ main1029857.shtml (accessed October 11, 2006).

2. Nanci Hellmich and Jo dee Black, "Desktop dining: recipe for disaster" *Great Falls Tribune Online Health*, March 1, 2004, www.greatfallstribune.com/news/stories/20040301/localnews/ 49568.html (accessed August 2006).

3. Donald R. Morse and M. L. Furst, "Meditation: An In-depth Study," *Journal of the American Society of Psychosomatic Dentistry and Medicine* 29, no. 5 (1982): 1–96.

4. Herbert Benson, *The Relaxation Response* (New York: William Morrow, 1975).

5. Deborah Kesten, *Feeding the Body, Nourishing the Soul: Essentials of Eating for Physical, Emotional, and Spiritual Well-Being* (Berkeley, CA: Conari Press, 1997).

6. Urasenke Foundation, "The Urasenke Tradition of Chado" (Kyoto, Japan: Urasenke Foundation, 1995).

7. G. D. Jacobs, "The Physiology of Mind-Body Interactions: The Stress Response and the Relaxation Response," *Journal of Alternative and Complementary Medicine* 8, no. 2 (2002): supplement 1: S8392.

8. R. J. Davidson, "Alterations in Brain and Immune Function Produced by Mindfulness Meditation," *Psychosomatic Medicine* 66, no. 1 (2004): 147–52.

9. Jean Kristeller, "An Exploratory Study of a Meditation-Based Intervention for Binge Eating Disorder," *Journal of Health Psychology* 4, no. 3 (1999): 357–63.

10. Jean Kristeller, "Know Your Hunger," *Spirituality & Health* 8, no. 2 (March/April 2005).

11. J. J. Daubenmier, G. Weidner, M. Sumner, N. Mendell, et al., "The Contribution of Changes in Diet, Exercise, and Stress Management to Changes in Coronary Risk in Women and Men in the Multisite Cardiac Lifestyle Intervention Program," *Annals of Behavioral Medicine* 33 (January 2007).

12. Gerdi Weidner (PhD, vice president and director of research, Preventive Medicine Research Institute, Sausalito, CA), in discussion with Deborah Kesten, October 20, 2006.

13. Ibid.

Chapter 4: Emotional Eating

1. Barbara Birsinger (PhD in theology, registered dietitian), in discussion with Deborah Kesten for six hours, during the week of September 26, 2006.

2. Cassandra Vieten (PhD, clinical psychologist and research scientist, San Francisco and Petaluma, CA), in discussion with Deborah Kesten, February 8, 2005.

3. Judith J. Wurtman, *Managing Your Mind and Mood through Food* (New York: Rawson Associates, 1986).

4. Eckhart Tolle, *The Power of Now* (Novato, CA: New World Library, 1999).

5. Vieten, February 8, 2005.

6. Overeaters Anonymous, www.oa.org/lifeline_monthly.html (accessed December 8, 2006).

7. Birsinger, September 26, 2006.

8. Barbara Birsinger, "Abstract: Effects of an Integrative Approach on Restoring Balance to Eating and Weight Issues" (Fair Grove, MO: Holos University Graduate Seminary, February 2006).

9. Instruments Barbara Birsinger used for pre- and postintervention tests include:

    (1) Intuitive Eating Scale (IES), 26 items: measures intrinsic eating, extrinsic eating, antidieting behaviors, and self-care practices. Hala Madanat, Jaylyn Hawks, and Ashley Harris, "The Intuitive Eating Scale: Development and Preliminary Validation," *American Journal of Health Education* 35, no. 2 (March/April 2004): 90.

    (2) Motivation for Eating Scale (MES), 43 items: measures the following subscales in relation to motivation for eating— emotional, physical, and environmental. Steven Hawks, Cari Merrill, Julie Gast, and Jaylyn Hawks, *Ecology of Food and Nutrition* 43 (2004): 307–26.

    (3) Dutch Eating Behavior Questionnaire (DEBQ), 33 items: measures restrained, emotional, and external eating behaviors. T. Van Strien, J. E. R. Fritjers, G. P. A. Bergers, and P. B. Defares, "The Dutch Eating Behavior Questionnaire for Assessment of Restrained, Emotional, and External Eating Behavior," *International Journal of Eating Disorders* 5 (1986): 295–315.

(4) Eating Attitudes Test (EAT), 26 items: screening measure for eating pathology. D. Garner et al., "Eating Attitudes Test," *Psychological Medicine* 12, no. 4 (1982): 71–78.

(5) Spiritual Well-Being Scale (SWBS), 20 items: measures subscales of existential and religious spiritual well-being. Craig W. Ellison, "Toward an Integrative Measure of Health and Well-Being," *Journal of Psychology and Theology* 19, no. 1 (1991): 35–48.

(6) Rosenberg Self-Esteem Scale (RSES), 10 items: measures general feelings of self-esteem. M. Rosenberg, *Society and the Adolescent Self-Image* (Middletown, CT: Wesleyan University Press, 1965).

(7) Body Satisfaction Scale (BSS), 21 items: measures the satisfaction with one's physical appearance. E. Stice, "A Prospective Test of the Dual Pathway Model of Bulimic Pathology: Mediating Effects of Dieting and Negative Affect," *Journal of Abnormal Psychology* 110 (2001): 124–35.

(8) Bem Sex Role Inventory (BSRI), 60 items: measures whether one has a masculine or feminine orientation. S. L. Bem, "The Measurement of Psychological Androgeny," *Journal of Clinical and Consulting Psychology* 42 (1974): 155–62.

(9) Body Mass Index (BMI): measures one's height and weight relationship to assess whether a person is overweight or obese.

(10) Food Habits Questionnaire (developed by Barbara Birsinger; qualitative dietary intake).

10. Barbara Birsinger, "Conversations with Bod: Discovering the Spiritual Archetypal and Symbolic Messages in Food, Eating, Body Language, and Weight" workshop, "Weekly Topics—Intended Results, Methods, and Measures," 2005.

11. Judith Wurtman, *Managing Mind and Mood Through Food* (New York: Perennial/HarperCollins, 1988).

12. Elizabeth Somer and Nancy Snyderman, *Food and Mood: The Complete Guide to Eating Well and Feeling Your Best* (New York: Henry Holt, 1996).

Chapter 5: Fast Foodism

1. Mark Hyman, "Systems Biology: The Gut-Brain-Fat Cell Connection and Obesity," editorial, *Alternative Therapies* 12, no. 1 (January/February 2006): 10.

2. Judith C. Rodriguez, "Fast Foods Health," *Gale Encyclopedia of Nutrition and Well Being* (New York: Gale Group, 2004), www.healthline.com/galecontent/fast-foods (accessed June 15, 2007).

3. James J. Ferguson, "Definition of Terms Used in the National Organic Program" (Gainesville: University of Florida, Institute of Food and Agricultural Sciences [UF/IFAS], Horticultural Sciences Department, Florida Cooperative Extension Service, January 2004), www.edis.ifas.ufl.edu/HS209 (accessed May 1, 2007).

4. "Junk food definition," Yourdictionary.com, www.yourdictionary.com/ahd/j/j0084300.html (accessed June 11, 2007).

5. William Saleian, "It's a Fat, Fat, Fat, Fat World," *San Francisco Chronicle*, September 17, 2006, E3; David Goldstein, "Junk-Food Makers Face FTC Scrutiny," *San Francisco Chronicle*, November 18, 2006, A8; Kim Severson, "Sugar Coated: We're Drowning in High Fructose Corn Syrup," *San Francisco Chronicle*, February 18, 2004, E6.

6. Bridget Murray, "Fast-Food Culture Serves Up Super-Size Americans," *Monitor on Psychology* 32, no. 11 (December 2001), www.apa.org/monitor/dec01/fastfood.html (accessed June 15, 2007).

7. Robert H. Lustig, "Childhood Obesity: Behavioral Aberration or Biochemical Drive? Reinterpreting the First Law of Thermodynamics," *Nature Clinical Practice Endocrinology & Metabolism* 8 (2006): 447–58.

8. "McDonald's USA Ingredients Listing for Popular Menu Items," www.mcdonalds.com/app_controller.nutrition.categories. ingredients.index.html (accessed January 13, 2007).

9. "Sugar: Sweet by Nature," advertisement, *News Tribune* (Tacoma, WA), December 7, 2006.

10. Michael F. Roizen and Mehmet C. Oz, "Food Fight: The Ghrelin versus Leptin Grudge Match," *You: On a Diet* (New York: Free Press, 2006).

11. Thomas Leuck and Kim Severson, "New York Bans Most Trans Fats in Restaurants," *New York Times*, December 6, 2006, www.nytimes.com/2006/12/06nyrefgion/06fat.html (accessed December 6, 2006); Georgia Jones, "Fast Foods! A 4-H Lifelong Learning Resource," *Journal of Nutrition Education and Behavior*, Society for Nutrition Education 38, no. 4 (July/August 2006): supplement S37; Bonnie Liebman, "The Pressure to Eat," *Nutrition Action* (July/August 1998), www.cspinet.org/nah/7_98eat.htm (accessed June 15, 2007); "Fast Food," Wikipedia, www.en.wikipedia.org/wiki/Fast_food (accessed December 5, 2006); D. Mozaffarian, M. B. Katan, A. Ascherio, M. M. Stampfer, and W. C. Willett, "Trans Fatty Acids and Cardiovascular Disease," *New England Journal of Medicine* 354, no. 15 (April 2006): 1601–13; F. B. Hu, R. M. van Dam, and S. Liu, "Diet and Risk of Type II Diabetes: The Role of Types of Fat and Carbohydrate," *Diabetologia* 44, no. 7 (July 2001): 805–17; R. M. van Dam, M. Stampfer, W. C. Willett, F. B. Hu, and E. B. Rimm, "Dietary Fat and Meat Intake in Relation to Risk of Type 2 Diabetes in Men," *Diabetes Care* 25, no. 3 (2002): 417–24; Anna Gosline, "Why Fast Foods Are Bad, Even in Moderation," *New Scientist*

(June 12, 2006), www.newscientist.com/article.ns?id=dn9318&f
eed1d=online-news_rss20 (accessed June 15, 2007).

12. Connie Guttersen, "America's Supersized Waistlines," *Foodservice: Recent Findings,* www.calolive.org/foodservice/findings/ findings_2003q1.html (accessed December 2, 2006); Leanie Lerche Davis, "Fast Food Creates Fat Kids," WebMD: Medical News Archives (January 5, 2004), www.webmd.com/content/ article/79/96083.htm (accessed December 6, 2006); Robert H. Lustig, "Childhood Obesity," 447–58; "WHO-MONICA Project: Risk Factors," abstract, *International Journal of Epidemiology* 18 (1989), supplement 1: S46–55.

13. G. Ma, Y. Li, Y. Wu, F. Zhai, Z. Cui, X. Hu, et al., "The Prevalence of Body Overweight and Obesity and Its Changes among Chinese People during 1992 to 2002," *Chinese Journal of Preventive Medicine* 39 (2005): 311–15 (in Chinese, with English abstract); Y. Wu, G. Ma, Y. Hu, Y. Li, X. Li, Z. Cui, et al., "The Current Prevalence Status of Body Overweight and Obesity in China: Data from the China Nutrition and Health Survey," *Chinese Journal of Preventive Medicine* 39 (2005): 316–20 (in Chinese, with English abstract).

14. Dean Ornish, *Eat More, Weigh Less: Dr. Dean Ornish's Life Choice Program for Losing Weight Safely while Eating Abundantly* (New York: HarperCollins, 1993).

15. Julie Meyer, "10 Best Slimming Foods," *Woman's Day* (October 3, 2006), 96.

Chapter 6: Solo Dining

1. The National Center on Addiction and Substance Abuse (CASA) at Columbia University, www.casacolumbia.org (accessed November 9, 2007).

2. M. W. Gillman, S. L. Rifas-Shiman, L. A. Frazier, and H. R. H. Rockette, "Family Dinner and Diet Quality among Older Children and Adolescents," *Archives of Family Medicine* 9 (March 2000): 235–40.

3. Richard S. Strauss and Harold A. Pollack, "Epidemic Increase in Childhood Overweight, 1986–1998," *Journal of the American Medical Association* 286, no. 22 (December 12, 2001): 2845–48.

4. Stewart Wolf and John G. Bruhn, *The Power of Clan: The Influence of Human Relationships on Heart Disease* (New Brunswick, NJ: Transaction, 1993).

5. Robert M. Nerem, Murina J. Levesque, and J. Fredrick Cornhill, "Social Environment as a Factor in Diet-Induced Atherosclerosis," *Science* New Series, 208, no. 4451 (June 27, 1980): 1475–76.

6. Marion Cunningham, in discussion with Deborah Kesten, April 2003.

7. Vinita Azarow, in discussion with Deborah Kesten, about her after-school meals made by Nonna, her Italian grandmother.

8. "Dream Dinners: Where Wonderful Meals Come True," www.dreamdinners.com (accessed January 3, 2007).

Chapter 7: Unappetizing Atmosphere

1. Elsie M. Widdowson, "Mental Contentment and Physical Growth," *The Lancet* 1, no. 24 (June 16, 1951): 1316–18.

2. Reginald Horsman, *Frontier Doctor William Beaumont, America's First Great Medical Scientist* (Columbia: University of Missouri Press, 1996).

3. Candace B. Pert, *Molecules of Emotion: The Science Behind Mind-Body Medicine; Why You Feel the Way You Feel* (New York: Scribner, 1997), 297–98.

4. N. Garg, B. Wansink, and Ji Jeffrey, "The Influence of Incidental Affect on Consumers' Food Intake," *Journal of Marketing* 71, no. 1 (January 2007), 194.

5. Marc Schweitzer, et al., "Healing Spaces: Elements of Environmental Design That Make an Impact on Health," *The Journal of Alternative and Complementary Medicine* 10 (2004), supplement 1: S71–S83.

6. Christine Aaron in conversation with author Mireille Guiliano and Oprah Winfrey, "Anti-Aging Breakthroughs," transcript, *Oprah: The Oprah Winfrey Show*, May 17, 2005 (Livingston, NJ: Burrelle's Information Services), 21.

Chapter 8: Sensory Disregard

1. Mark Morford, "Obese American Tourists, Ho!" Notes & Errata, *San Francisco Chronicle*, February 22, 2006, www.sfgate.com/ cgi-bin/article.cgi?f=/gate/archive/2006/02/22/notes022206. DTL&nl=fix (accessed June 15, 2007).

2. Seth Roberts, "What Makes Food Fattening? A Pavlovian Theory of Weight Control" (unpublished theory article, University of California, Berkeley, February 2005), 1–77.

3. "Instant Willpower!" *Woman's World* 27, no. 40 (October 3, 2006), 18–19.

4. Seth Roberts, *The Shangri-La Diet* (New York: Putnam, 2006).

5. Keri Brenner, "Dissecting the Shangri-La Diet Fad," *The Olympian*, July 31, 2006, B8.

6. Hildegard of Bingen, *Secrets of God: Writings of Hildegard of Bingen*, ed. Sabrina Flanagan (Boston: Shambhala, 1996).

7. Barbara Birsinger, "Conversations with Bod" workshop, "Weekly Topics—Intended Results, Methods, and Measures," 2005.

8. Birsinger, September 26, 2006.

9. Namgyal Qusar, First International Conference on Tibetan Medicine, Washington, D.C., November 7–9, 1998.

10. Michael Mayer, (PhD, psychologist, Orinda, CA), in discussion with Deborah Kesten, December 5, 1996.

Chapter 9: Enlightened Exercise

1. Bruce Heller in discussion with Deborah Kesten, January 30, 2007.

2. Bruce Milliman, in discussion with Deborah Kesten, January 26, 2007.

3. Heller, January 30, 2007.

4. Ibid.

5. Ibid.

6. Ibid.

7. W. C. Miller, D. M. Koceja, and E. J. Hamilton, "A Meta-Analysis of the Past 25 Years of Weight Loss Research Using Diet, Exercise or Diet Plus Exercise Intervention," *International Journal of Obesity* 21, no. 10 (October 1997): 941–47.

8. Peg Jordan, *The Fitness Instinct: The Revolutionary New Approach to Healthy Exercise That Is Fun, Natural, and No Sweat* (Emmaus, PA: Rodale Books, 2000); WebMD Live Events Transcript Archive, "Exercise: Get Going and Keep Going—Meg Jordan, PhD, RN," January 21, 2003, www.webmd.com/content/article/60/66933.htm (accessed February 2, 2007).

9. USDA: United States Department of Agriculture, "Inside the Pyramid: What Is Physical Activity?" MyPyramid.gov, www.mypyramid.gov/pyramid/physical_activity.html (accessed February 2, 2007).

Chapter 10: In Action

1. Mireille Guiliano, author presentation, Book Passage, Corde Madera, CA, November 11, 2006; Mireille Guiliano, *French Women Don't Get Fat: The Secret of Eating for Pleasure* (New York: Knopf, 2005); Christine Aaron in conversation with author Mireille Guiliano and Oprah Winfrey, "Anti-Aging Breakthroughs, *Oprah: The Oprah Winfrey Show*, May 17, 2005.

2. Ibid.

Index

About the Authors

Deborah Kesten, MPH, is an international nutrition researcher and educator, with a specialty in preventing and reversing obesity and heart disease. She was the nutritionist on Dr. Dean Ornish's first clinical trial for reversing heart disease through lifestyle changes, and co-principal investigator on research about her Whole Person Nutrition Model and Program, the results of which were published in *Explore: The Journal of Science and Healing*. With more than two hundred published nutrition and health articles, she is also the award-winning author of *Feeding the Body, Nourishing the Soul* and *The Healing Secrets of Food*, a comprehensive, evidence-based nutrition program about the power of food to heal multidimensionally. Among Kesten's accomplishments are contributions to scientific books and medical journals, including the *Journal of the American Medical Association*. She lives in the state of Washington with her husband, Larry Scherwitz, PhD.

Larry Scherwitz, PhD, is an international research scientist who has specialized in mind-body research and lifestyle and their link to preventing and reversing heart disease and obesity. His extensive experience initiating and directing comprehensive, sustainable, lifestyle-change programs with heart patients and their families includes directing seven lifestyle programs (four in the United States, three in Europe). Dr. Scherwitz's research has been published in a plethora of prestigious medical journals, including the *Journal of the American Medical Association* and *The Lancet*. He has also been director of research and co-principal investigator with Dean Ornish, MD, on his heart disease reversal research. Presently, he is director of clinical sciences at the American Institute of Biosocial and Medical Research (AIBMR) Life Sciences, Inc., in Washington. He is married to Deborah Kesten, MPH.

Visit them at their website, www.EnlightenedDiet.com.